PRAISE FOR *THE HIGHLY SENSITIVE MAN*

"Tom Falkenstein's outstanding book contains a thorough review of all the relevant scientific studies and literature, many innovative and new techniques for the highly sensitive man to cope with overstimulation, fascinating stories by sensitive men and practical tips to increase their self-worth and self-acceptance. This book is a masterpiece that every sensitive man should read."

TED ZEFF, PHD, author of *The Strong Sensitive Boy,*
The Highly Sensitive Person's Survival Guide and
The Power of Sensitivity

"A book that all highly sensitive people should read! Carefully and meticulously crafted ... rooted in the rigorous science of sensory processing sensitivity ... [this book] provides numerous ways we can grow into our own skins as people who experience the world slightly differently. A powerful and ennobling addition to every highly sensitive person's library!"

TRACY COOPER, PHD, author of *Thrill!: The High*
Sensation Seeking Highly Sensitive Person

"This book not only shows why highly sensitive men are particularly suffering in the current masculinity crisis, but also why they have exactly the right qualities to turn this crisis into an opportunity. It's an important book that relieves the pressure of being a highly sensitive man and offers practical tools to the reader. Thank you, Tom Falkenstein."

GEORG PARLOW, author of *Highly Sensitive*

"Tom Falkenstein's book is characterized by a clear, precise, and practical style. It's a unique and encouraging book for all of those men who want to understand and use their sensitive temperament better."

BRIGITTE SCHORR, author of *Highly Sensitive in Relationships*

"*The Highly Sensitive Man* is a major contribution to the expansion of mental, physical, emotional, and soulful intelligence. Tom Falkenstein has written a book that cracks open the conversation about how men can blend their strength, sensitivity, and unique gifts into a more modern and whole definition of what it is to be a man. It's a breath of fresh air in the midst of a cultural determination to reduce toxic masculinity. This book is a balm, a movement, and a revelation … The integrating of the knowledge in this book would allow for a complete cultural sea change around what it is to be a man."

ALANIS MORISSETTE, singer and songwriter

TOM FALKENSTEIN

The Highly Sensitive Man

Finding Strength in Sensitivity

Thorsons

The reader is advised that this book is not intended to be a substitute
for an assessment by, and advice from, an appropriate medical professional(s).
This book contains general information regarding high sensitivity and
should be viewed as purely educational in nature.

Thorsons
An imprint of HarperCollins*Publishers*
1 London Bridge Street
London SE1 9GF

www.harpercollins.co.uk

German language edition © 2017 by Junfermann Verlag.
English translation by Ben Fergusson. This translation published by
arrangement with Agence Schweiger.

English language edition first published in the US by
Citadel Press Books, Kensington Publishing Corp. 2019
This Thorsons edition published 2019

1 3 5 7 9 10 8 6 4 2

A catalogue record of this book is
available from the British Library

ISBN 978-0-00-836644-5

Printed and bound in Great Britain by
CPI Group (UK) Ltd, Croydon

MIX
Paper from
responsible sources
FSC
www.fsc.org   FSC™ C007454

This book is produced from independently certified FSC™ paper
to ensure responsible forest management.

For more information visit: www.harpercollins.co.uk/green

For Ben and Theo

Contents

This excessive sensitiveness very often brings an enrichment of the personality and contributes more to its charm than to the undoing of a person's character. Only, when difficult and unusual situations arise, the advantage frequently turns into a very great disadvantage, since calm consideration is then disturbed by untimely affects. Nothing could be more mistaken, though, than to regard this excessive sensitiveness as in itself a pathological character component. If that were really so, we should have to rate about one quarter of humanity as pathological.

A certain innate sensitiveness produces a special prehistory, a special way of experiencing infantile events, which in their turn are not without influence on the development of the child's view of the world. Events bound up with powerful impressions can never pass off without leaving some trace on sensitive people. Some of them remain effective throughout life, and such events can have a determining influence on a person's whole mental development.

—CARL JUNG, on particularly
sensitive people, 1913

Foreword

I REALLY LIKE SENSITIVE MEN just because of those two words. First, they are men and I usually like being with men. Second, they are highly sensitive. To me, that means I can have deep conversations with them. Superficial small talk is *so* boring for the highly sensitive. These men have ideas. But they are also usually better listeners than the average man. They often show warmth and empathy. If you dig down, not far, you find they have a spiritual vein. They are generally ethical in their behavior and nonviolent. They are never perfect, trust me on that, but that's good, too.

So I like that combination: sensitive man. If you are reading this, I assume that those words describe you or someone you care about. This book is about joining those two words in your mind, as a wonderful thing, just as I join them.

If *you* are a sensitive man, please make that leap to valuing yourself, not only for yourself but also for the rest of us. We really, really, really need you. We need you to find ways to influence the world because you have what it takes—deep ideas, the ability to find the best strategies, empathy for others, and ethics. But we want you to do it in the right way for you. And we want you to do whatever healing you need and to stay grounded in your center, to not be overstimulated. There's no need to burn out. Nothing is helped in the long run by that. You need to keep renewing your equanimity, meaning your wisdom, and this book is a treasure trove of ways to do that.

About your author: The minute I met Tom Falkenstein in 2015 I liked him. Getting to know him just a little more, I saw that Tom had everything needed to write this book: he has a good grasp of the science behind sensitivity and enough training and experience to have a wealth of practical ideas. Above all, he is a licensed clinician, meaning, among many other things, that he can tell sensitivity from psychological disorders. Sometimes highly sensitive people are misdiagnosed and do not have a disorder. Sometimes highly sensitive people can have a disorder. And sometimes a person will want to think the only problem is sensitivity, when there is actually something else there and the person is not highly sensitive at all. Tom understands all of this and will impart that to you as well.

Given all of this, I have been happy to help him in any way I could with this book. We had several video calls, Berlin to San Francisco. He asked good questions, and I think we enjoyed ourselves, too. Working with him, I found I trusted him, and I wish you could meet him, too. But I am sure his author's voice will come across to you as warm, authentic, knowledgeable, and experienced—highly sensitive, perhaps like you.

—*Elaine Aron*
San Francisco

Introduction

"I HATE THAT I'M SO sensitive!" My client, a man in his mid twenties, was sitting across from me and had just clearly expressed how and why he felt so angry. It was the first warm day in London that spring, and suddenly the room was completely still. This young man had been coming to the clinic for some time and was being treated for recurrent depression. I was his psychotherapist, and over the course of his treatment, we kept indirectly coming back to the topic of sensitivity. But this was the first time that he had openly identified himself as sensitive and the first time that he had revealed the self-hatred he felt about his sensitivity. It was, for him, a painful but important step in dealing with his sensitive temperament, which he had struggled with since he was a child. For me, it was a key moment in my professional career because this client had clearly identified something that I had encountered countless times over the years in my work without, until that moment, having had a name for it or being able to concretely identify the phenomenon—the highly sensitive man.

During my postgraduate training in psychotherapy in Berlin, I kept coming across a particular type of client that I experienced as particularly sensitive, thoughtful, intuitive, conscientious, often introverted, and sometimes shy. These clients came to therapy for the most varied reasons: depression, anxiety, relationship problems. But they all shared an underlying characteristic: they were very sensitive, and because of this, they experienced their internal and external worlds in a very subtle and perceptive way.

After a while, I realized that I particularly enjoyed working with this group of clients, precisely because of the way that they perceived and dealt with the world. But it also became increasingly clear to me that it was my male, rather than my female clients who had the greatest problems with the sensitivity that they described and who in therapy often expressed a desire to be less sensitive. Again and again, I saw the huge amount of psychological suffering caused by the discrepancy between how these men were and how they thought a man *should* be. They often felt shame and a sense of inferiority about their sensitive disposition, which had been part of their lives since childhood, and they saw their sensitivity as "unmanly," "feminine," and "unattractive." Many had tried for a long time to deny their sensitivity or to hide it from others—nearly always in vain. The conviction that being sensitive meant that you couldn't be manly seemed deeply rooted.

During my sessions, I constantly heard male clients saying that they wished they were tougher, more physically and mentally resilient, and that they wished they could learn to be more extroverted in social situations. They usually thought that it was this that would make them more successful in their jobs and more attractive to potential partners. Often these men also wanted to have less-conflicted relationships with their own fathers and with other men. Essentially, though, it always came back to the same basic idea: they wanted to be more like what they saw as a "typical man." And this typical man was not particularly sensitive.

At that time, I hadn't yet come across the concept of high sensitivity as an innate temperamental trait (i.e., a characteristic that you are born with) and wasn't aware of the extensive research done regarding the highly sensitive person (HSP) by the clinical psychologist Elaine Aron, Ph.D., and her colleagues. She has been researching this concept since the early 1990s, when she began to look into the concept of "innate sensitivity" in certain people. It was a concept that Carl Jung, the Swiss psychiatrist and founder of analytical psychology, had described as early as 1913. With my interest piqued by my experiences in London, I began to read more and more about human sensitivity and discovered the concept of sensory processing sensitivity, as high sensitivity is called in academic research. I had the feeling that I had come across a groundbreaking psychological concept that was going to have a huge impact on my work as a therapist. The idea that people are born with different sensitivities that affect the way that they react to the world around them seemed to explain so many things I had seen in my practice. So over the next few years, I immersed myself in all of the available material on high sensitivity and began a dialogue with Elaine Aron, who gave me an in-depth personal insight into her research and her therapeutic work with highly sensitive patients.

As I began to investigate the subject of high sensitivity more deeply, I really struggled to find books that described the specific challenges of high sensitivity from a male perspective. The majority of books on high sensitivity were written by women and seemed to be primarily aimed at female readers. Yet in my psychotherapeutic practice and my consultancy work, I saw that it was particularly men who struggled with being highly sensitive. And although a few self-help books touch on the difficulties that sensitive men experience when trying to live up to traditional ideas about masculinity in Western culture, there is still no book that really focuses on the topic of highly sensitive masculinity, which, of course, only exacerbates the taboo around it. That's what I want to change with this book.

It is important to me that this book contributes to the long-neglected issue of empowerment for highly sensitive men because I believe that their role in the world is very important and that it comes with many challenges and opportunities. I consider the high sensitivity of many men to be a completely essential part of masculine identity and something that can enrich the lives of these men and the lives of others. Sensitivity is in no way a shameful or "unmanly" flaw that one has to get over.

To see the opportunities that your sensitivity offers you, however, you have to learn to deal well and responsibly with it. You have to accept it, learn to value it, and use it positively in your relationships with other people. When this happens, I believe that a highly sensitive disposition can make men particularly good fathers, husbands, partners, son, brothers, and friends.

At the same time, I think it's important to say that your high sensitivity—once you've detected it and identified it—should not be used as an excuse to avoid doing things that you actually just don't want to do. I also believe that it is not something to become arrogant or boastful about, in the sense of "I'm special, because I'm so sensitive." High sensitivity is a completely neutral disposition, an innate temperamental trait.[1] Having a highly sensitive disposition is not automatically a good thing nor is it a bad thing. It is, of course, an important part of your personality, but at the end of the day it is exactly that—one part, one aspect of your complex personal makeup. I thus feel that it's problematic to reduce yourself to that one quality or to wear your highly sensitive nature like a badge of honor. I see highly sensitive men as neither "delicate flowers" nor as "golden children."

In my work with highly sensitive clients, I often compare a highly sensitive disposition to being born with very fair skin. You can complain that you weren't born with darker skin, and you might be envious of friends who are able to sun themselves on the beach, in the garden, or in the park and not worry about burning. But at the end of the day, you have to accept that your skin is different. It's not better, not worse, just different. People with very fair skin can also go sunbathing if they want; they just can't stay in the sun for as long as other people. They also have to take different precautions, such as using high SPF sunscreen, finding somewhere shady to sit, and wearing a hat or light-colored clothing. In fact, people with pale skin can enjoy the "sunny" moments in life just as much as anyone else; they just have to learn how to do it in their own and sometimes a slightly different way. And that's the crux of the matter: to accept the situation as it actually is and, ultimately, to find your own individual and authentic way of learning to live with it.

There has been a sharp increase in the number of publications on and academic research into high sensitivity over the last few years. Through this, the term *high sensitivity* is becoming increasingly well recognized internationally. My guess is that this also has something to do with the time in which we currently live. I notice that many people feel that their personal lives and their careers are increasingly fast paced and achievement oriented, and they often feel constantly stressed, exhausted, overstimulated, and under nonstop pressure. The line dividing our private and public lives continues to become more and more blurred, and Western society increasingly seems to celebrate and demand that we cultivate personality traits that aren't normally associated with sensitive, introverted, and reserved people.

What is increasingly valued is the ability to push on through, to work quickly and make quick decisions, to be able to do many things at once, and to appear self-confident and extroverted in front of groups of people—whether it's with other children in the kindergarten or primary school or with other adults in the workplace. Added to this is the value placed on making a good first impression, the pressure to be constantly available via email and cell phone, and the ability to present yourself well, whether on social media or in real life. Many psychologists and psychiatrists have gone as far as labeling this as an "epidemic of narcissism"[2] in what they term a "narcissistic society."

It would seem, in the West, that more and more value is being placed on behaviors and qualities that highly sensitive people either often find more difficult to access or that make them feel overstimulated or exhausted. And yet these are the very qualities and positive characteristics of many highly sensitive people—a high capacity for empathy, emotional depth, and subtlety, a tendency to deal with things in an ethical way, and a finely tuned sense of perception—that seem more important now than ever before if we are going to be able to deal with the social and economic challenges of our world.

I believe that dealing with your own specific sensitivity in a natural and authentic way is not just vital for every single man but also vital for society as a whole. If highly sensitive men are able to live in harmony with their temperaments, to use their skills actively and positively, and to no longer feel ashamed about them, hide them, or believe that they make them inferior as people, then they can profoundly change the relationship that they have with themselves. But this will also change their relationship with other people, whether family, friends, or colleagues, and this could have far-reaching consequences. Because, through this, society's conception of what it means to be a man could change. We could have a less rigid, less narrow, freer, more complex understanding of masculinity. The result of this change, which is already happening, could be a more realistic and more authentic male image, so that being manly *and* being sensitive no longer seem to be mutually exclusive. I believe that sensitive men in particular could drive this change and even lead it, but they can only do so if they have accepted their own high sensitivity and can sense that they are important, not just for the evolution of men but also of society as a whole.

This book is written in two parts: theory and practice. In the first part of the book, I will use theoretical concepts from the fields of psychology and medicine to discuss how we see men in contemporary Western society and the unique problems they are currently facing. I will illuminate the negative effects that a traditional, antiquated image of men can have and explain why it is highly sensitive men in particular who have the power to bring about necessary change and who thus have huge social value. I will then give you an overview of how the concept of high sensitivity was developed and describe exactly what high sensitivity is, as well as what it is not, and how you can tell whether you yourself are highly sensitive. You will learn what the typical characteristics of highly sensitive men are, but also how being highly sensitive can be both a challenge and an asset. And you will also learn to differentiate high sensitivity from psychological disorders.

In the second half of the book, I will give you practical tools that will help you deal with the challenges of being highly sensitive and the situations that highly sensitive people often find difficult. I will show you how you can fundamentally improve the quality of your everyday life through emotional regulation, mindfulness, acceptance, relaxation, self-compassion, and self-care. And I'll show you the best way of putting these techniques into practice. I will offer you concrete exercises and numerous strategies that have been particularly helpful to my highly sensitive clients over the years.

Each chapter is also followed by a conversation with a highly sensitive man. In these sections, the men describe what effect their high sensitivity has had on their careers, their sexuality, and their relationships, and how they've learned to deal with its downsides and get the most out of their disposition. The book ends with a conversation between Elaine Aron and myself about the key role that highly sensitive men have in the world today.

As a cognitive behavioral psychotherapist, it is, of course, in my nature to ask you to reflect on many questions over the course of this book, rather than just giving you a set of directives to follow. In doing so, I hope to spark off a process in which you begin to deal with your sensitivity in a very personal way. Once you have read this book, my hope is that you will feel more able to accept yourself as a highly sensitive man, exactly as you are, and that you will have learned to better look after yourself in your daily life. It would make me particularly happy if, through reading this book, any lingering feeling of being "not quite right" diminishes and that you learn to like your sensitive side more. Although I am aware of the limits of self-help books, I also believe in the power of books, which often leave behind subtle but far-reaching traces in us.

PART I

The Phenomenon of High Sensitivity

A Turning Point in Masculinity: The Importance of Highly Sensitive Men in Society

H AS THE TIME COME FOR male emancipation? And if so, then what would that emancipation look like? While feminism is experiencing its "fourth wave," men seem to be having a much harder time dealing with themselves and their place in society. And yet anyone who follows current trends in the media will have noticed that questions around male identity and role models and men's psychological well-being have been an increasingly common topic of discussion over the last few years. You only have to open a magazine or newspaper, turn on your TV, or open your browser to discover an ever-growing interest in stories about being a father, being a man, or how to balance a career with a family. Many of these articles have started talking about an apparent "crisis of masculinity."

The headlines for these articles attempt to address male identity, but often fall into the trap of sounding ironic and sometimes even sarcastic and critical: "Men in Crisis: Time to Pull Yourselves Together,"[1] "The Weaker Sex,"[2] "Crisis in Masculinity: Who is the Stronger Sex?"[3] and "Search for Identity: Super-Dads or Vain Peacocks"[4] are just a few examples. They all seem to agree to some extent that there is a crisis. But reading these articles, one gets the impression that no one really knows how to even start dealing with the problem, let alone what a solution to it might look like. One also gets the impression from these articles that we need to keep any genuine sympathy for these "poor men" in check: the patriarchy is still just too dominant to allow ourselves that luxury.

In this chapter, I want to begin by dealing with the question of how men are really doing in Western societies and to bring in some opinions and studies from the United States, Europe, and beyond. Because this is a book about highly sensitive men, I think it's important that we clearly outline the social context in which men are currently living. This chapter is therefore, in the first instance, a plea for greater diversity in masculinity—a diversity I believe we need and that could represent a possible solution to our so-called "crisis of masculinity." I'm also convinced that highly sensitive men have a key role to play in this long-overdue emancipation of men from classic stereotypes of masculinity, precisely because they challenge and therefore expand our image of the "typical strong man."

Is Masculinity in Crisis?

Though it was founded in 1901, it took the renowned British Psychological Society until 2014 to dedicate a whole issue of its journal, *The Psychologist*, to the psychological health of men.[5] This followed a series of discussions among politicians and in the media about an apparent "crisis of masculinity" that was raging in the country.[6] But this recent interest in the male psyche and in male identity isn't just a European phenomenon. In the United States, too, the term *toxic masculinity*, describing a particularly unhealthy form of male identity, has increasingly been doing the rounds.[7] Indeed, one of the most influential psychologists of our time, Philip Zimbardo—who gained international notoriety for his 1971 Stanford Prison Experiment—devoted his last book to the male identity crisis.[8] Toxic masculinity has also been addressed by British author Jack Urwin in his book *Man Up: Surviving Modern Masculinity*,[9] and in Germany, the magazine *Der Spiegel* published a column dedicated to the topic, titled "It's a Boy." The author, Margarete Stokowski, wrote, "There's an English term, 'toxic masculinity,' used to describe a form of masculinity based on dominance and violence that rejects emotions. It's a problem that boys and men are constantly told that 'real guys' don't cry, are highly, almost animalistically sexual, and crush anything that stands in their way. It's a problem for both men and women. This is the form of masculinity that we need to address. Just because it's widespread doesn't mean that it's natural."[10]

So it seems everyone is talking about a "crisis in masculinity." It is a crisis marked by men's insecurity about their role in society, their identity, their values, their sexuality, their careers, and their relationships.[1] At the same time, academics are telling us that "we know far less about the psychological and physical health of men than of women."[12] Why is this?

Michael Addis, a professor of psychology and a leading researcher into male identity and psychological health, has highlighted a deficit in our knowledge about men suffering from depression and argues that this has cultural, social, and historical roots. If we look at whether gender affects how people experience depression, how they express it, and how it's treated, it quickly becomes clear that *gender* has for a long time referred to women and not to men. According to Addis, this is because, socially and historically, men have been seen as the dominant group and thus representative of normal psychological health. Women have thus been understood as the nondominant group, which deviated from the norm, and they have been examined and understood from this perspective. One of the countless problems of this approach is that the experiences and specific challenges of the "dominant group," in this case men, have remained hidden.[13]

As we have discussed, though, this is finally beginning to change, with men's psychological health beginning to become part of our public discourse. What in the past was taken for granted is now being questioned. And perhaps it is precisely this questioning and the identification, analysis, and redefining that this entails, that is being understood as a crisis in masculinity and as a challenge to the "stronger sex."

How Are Men Doing?

While it is true that a higher percentage of women than men will be diagnosed with an anxiety disorder or a depressive episode, the suicide rate among men is much higher. In the United States, the suicide rate is notably higher in men than in women. According to data from the Centers for Disease Control and Prevention, men account for 77 percent of the forty-five thousand people who kill themselves every year in the United States. In fact, men commit suicide more than women everywhere in the world.[14] Men are more likely to suffer from addiction,[15] and when men discuss depressive symptoms with their doctor, they are less likely than women to be diagnosed with depression and consequently don't receive adequate therapeutic and pharmacological treatment.[16]

Young men are currently less academically successful at secondary school than young women. The number of men applying to university is now lower than the number of women applying,[17] and a far higher number of men drop out.[18] Men are also far more likely to be arrested. Ninety-three percent of people in prison are men.[19] These are startling numbers.

Even in wealthy industrialized nations, men die on average around five to ten years earlier than women. Although the causes are potentially manifold, medical opinion increasingly points to lifestyle, behavior, and environment, rather than biological difference, as being the most likely reasons behind this disparity between the sexes. Indeed, Dr. Thomas Perls, a professor at Boston University's School of Medicine, has been researching life expectancy for many years, and he believes that around 70 percent of this difference in life expectancy is due to lifestyle, behavior, and environment, with the remaining 30 percent being attributed to genetic or biological factors.[20] The conviction that lifestyle and behavior, rather than biological difference, are the reasons behind men dying earlier than women is also backed up by Dr. Marc Luy's "cloister study." His research shows that life expectancy among monks and nuns, who live in a nearly identical environment with a very similar lifestyle, is almost exactly the same. What's more, the monks who took part in the study lived on average around four years longer than men in the general population. Luy believes that the reasons for this difference are rooted in the monastic lifestyle, which is based on a daily routine that is consciously organized and highly regulated, a healthier lifestyle, and lower levels of stress.[21]

If behavior and lifestyle do indeed have such a decisive impact on men's psychological and physical health compared with simple biology, then this raises the question, What is influencing men's behavior and the sometimes self-destructive lifestyle that results from it? The answer, to a very great degree, appears to lie in the socialization of men and the "masculine" values and norms that men consequently internalize and then express in their behavior.

When Is a Man a Man?

If we take a moment to ask ourselves what makes a man "manly," that is to say, what the social expectations for men are, we will likely come up with different answers. I would assume, however, that many of us would name several classic, traditional masculine attributes: physical strength, stamina, emotional control, stoicism, independence, heterosexuality, drive, bravery, dominance, risk-taking, competitiveness, professional success, and sexual performance. In other words, we would probably describe, more or less, the typical image of the "strong man." I suspect that words such as *sensitive, emotional, delicate,* or *compassionate* would come up less often.

Of course, we have been talking about the "new man" for decades, embodied by the likes of "metrosexuals" and style-conscious figures like David Beckham. There is no question that society's ideas around male identity have changed over the past decades, and there are plenty of indicators to back this up. For instance, fathers now spend on average eight hours a week on childcare; this is three times as much as was reported in 1965. And they spend on average ten hours on household chores, up from four hours in 1965.[22] And yet our image of "new men" is still heavily influenced by those classic, traditional attributes: professional success, stamina, status, performance, self-control, and heterosexuality. This is backed up by numerous psychological studies over the last forty years that tell us that, despite huge social change, the stereotypical image of the "strong man" is still firmly with us at all ages, in all ethnic groups, and among all socio-economic backgrounds. In the face of problems, men tend not to seek out emotional or professional help from other people. They use, more often than women, alcohol or drugs to numb unpleasant feelings and, in crises, tend to try to deal with things on their own, instead of searching out closeness or help from others.[23] A new metrosexual masculinity that focuses simply on external appearance and the existence of paternity leave in many countries (ninety-two countries, but *not* the United States) have done very little to change this.

The socialization of men, so essential to their identity, lifestyle, and behavior, seems to be a decisive part of the problem. When we talk about socialization, we mean the process of integrating and adapting to the society and culture that surrounds us, through, for instance, the family, school, friends, the church, or the media. Early on in his life, a boy will begin to take on those gender-specific behaviors, attitudes, values, norms, and ideologies that the society in which he is growing up deems to be masculine and acceptable. The unfortunately still popular blue onesie is just the beginning of this process and is a public symbol of a socialization that often takes far more subtle forms.

We know, however, that the internalization of particularly restrictive socially masculine norms can have negative consequences on how a man feels.[24] This happens when he begins to feel that the way he *is* does not fit with the way he thinks he *should be*. We call this "gender role strain" and "gender role conflict." Both concepts are used to measure and describe the emotional stress and conflict that men feel when they suffer emotionally from internalizing restrictive and unachievable masculine norms.[25] Jim O'Neil, the psychology professor and pioneer who first described gender role conflict, described the concept as follows: "Gender role conflict (GRC) is defined as a psychological state in which socialized gender roles have negative consequences for the person or others."[26] Psychologist Michael Addis also uses this concept in his work, showing that it is precisely those men who have strongly internalized traditional masculine norms and values—such as self-sufficiency, strength, and independence—who have a higher risk of suffering from depressive episodes and are less likely to seek professional help to deal with them.[27] It seems that old but still active adages such as "boys don't cry" and men need to "keep a stiff upper lip" can actually be detrimental to men's physical and mental health. Certainly, all men could benefit from loosening the restraints put on them by traditional masculine norms and values, but unfortunately, the fear of not being manly enough holds them firmly in place.

The Fear of Not Being Manly Enough

O'Neil believes that men's fear of not appearing to be masculine enough—or even worse, feminine—is often the main source of the hard and rigid armor that men put on, or allow society to put on them. He argues that this fear of the feminine is connected to strong,

negative feelings that are related to stereotypes about feminine values, beliefs, and behaviors and that these stereotypes are formed
during our childhoods by parents, peers, and social norms. Men's
conscious and subconscious fear of the feminine has been a consistent theme in academic literature for years.[28]

I often observe this in my work with male clients—men who
quickly feel ashamed when they believe that they haven't behaved
in a way that, in their opinion, fits with the behavior of a "real man."
The process often begins in childhood. Shame is an intense emotion
and a powerful tool of socialization. When we feel ashamed, we
often connect this with a fear of being shut out, of no longer belong-
ing to a group. Among prehistoric societies, this was a matter of life
or death.

But when the internalization of traditional masculine values and
ideals has reached such a pitch that it has clear and grave psychological and physical consequences, when it even leads to men dying
earlier because they seek out medical help too late or are unaware
that they're even ill, when they won't ask for help or confide in anyone else, then it is surely high time that we question and broaden
our definitions of these traditional masculine values.

I believe that the highly sensitive man has a key role to play in
this, because his inborn high sensitivity and the emotionality and
subtlety of feeling that comes with it automatically challenge traditional masculine norms, values, and behaviors, such as hardness,
toughness, stamina, competitiveness, and self-control. And he does
this without necessarily being conscious of it. He does it just by
being himself. This is the vital role that the highly sensitive man can
play in society—challenging taboos around vulnerability, sensitivity,
empathy, and, in particular, emotionality. And all men can profit, be
they young or old, heterosexual or homosexual, highly sensitive or
not highly sensitive. If a more authentic, holistic, and multifaceted
form of masculinity could emerge because of this, a form that would
allow *all* men in society to be sensitive and emotional without having to feel shame, anxiety, or a sense of inferiority, then we all win.

What We Define as Masculine
is Not Set in Stone

Society's view of how a man should be and what attributes are desirable and attractive in him is something that is more flexible than
we think. In her book *A History of Male Psychological Illness in Britain:
1945–1980*, historian Allison Haggett, Ph.D., describes the development of men's psychological problems in the United Kingdom since
the Second World War.[29] When I talked to her, she explained to me
that she finds the current, very narrow definition of masculinity in
the Western world to be "problematic and restrictive," referencing
numerous psychological and medical studies on men's health.

Haggett also describes how our understanding of typical masculinity has changed radically throughout history and says that, from
a historical perspective, it is much harder to define than we might
suppose. In her book, she argues that masculine attributes are first
and foremost socially constructed and not biologically determined.
They are, therefore, prone to change and have often done so in the
past. She describes how, during the Georgian era (1714–1830), just before the start of the Industrial Revolution in Great Britain, the picture
of a desirable man was completely different from the image we have
today. At that time, masculinity was equated with wisdom and virtu-
ousness. Not only was it socially acceptable for a man to express
himself emotionally, it was positively desirable. The Georgian man
was not afraid of being scorned for showing emotion. According to
Haggett, this led to a culture of introspection among men, in which
it was socially acceptable to be self-reflective and contemplative.

The central nervous system was also seen as being particularly
important in understanding the human body at that time, and it was
believed that a particularly nervous or sensitive disposition was a
clear indication of a noble or educated background and refinement,
not a sign of a lack of masculinity. The finer and more sensitive a
man's nervous system was, the better. What we might now call
"weak nerves" used to be something that was valued.

Our understanding of masculinity was, however, profoundly changed by the new focus on productivity and efficiency during the Industrial Revolution and the twentieth century's two world wars. Since then, open displays of emotion by men, with the exception of anger, have been stigmatized and are commonly seen as something negative and embarrassing.[30]

In order for men to assert themselves socially and professionally, it became increasingly important in the Western world for them to develop characteristics such as dominance, independence, and high performance. But as we have seen in this chapter, men have paid a high price for this. The rest of society has paid, too: their partners, their families, their children, their siblings, their parents, and their friends. It has affected all of us.

It goes without saying that when I talk about men as a whole, I am generalizing and simplifying enormously. But let us allow ourselves to do just that for a moment so that we can create a picture of the symbiotic interdependence between the sexes. When the position of women in our society changes—which has particularly been the case since the feminist women's movement from the 1960s onward—then that has an effect on men and vice versa. A man who finds it difficult to recognize his own emotional needs and feelings, and who cannot express these fully to other people, will find relationships with other people difficult and won't be able to become an emotionally satisfying or emotionally available partner. A man who primarily defines his own self-worth through his professional success or has learned to only express emotional intimacy through his sexuality is just as problematic. Both of these personality aspects will have negative outcomes on his partners, his family, his relationships, his health, and his whole community. It is therefore in the interest of both men *and* women that men are better able to free themselves from the traditional values of masculinity. This will allow men to open up emotionally, to be seen as multifaceted, to be vulnerable, and to show their emotions without being scared of being shamed for being a "wimp" or a "sissy." Men and women both profit when they are able to live fully as complete equals—free, autonomous, self-confident, multilayered, and multifaceted, with space for personal growth.

Male Emancipation

So what might male emancipation look like? I don't believe that all men have to become more sensitive or somehow soften their appearance or their nature, nor do I think that we should be aiming to return to a Georgian ideal of masculinity that values the particular traits of the highly sensitive man. What I do believe is that we need to expand our idea of what masculinity can be and feel able to define it more freely, so that it includes every man and boy as he is, encompassing all of his unique facets, complexities, and contradictions. We need to stop reducing ourselves and being reduced by others. We need to stop seeing everything as black and white and start seeing the great spectrum of shades that exists among men. We need to stop saying "either-or" and start saying "as well as." Masculine and sensitive, masculine and emotional. And the more that the highly sensitive man is able to deal with and thrive with his high sensitivity, to live with it with more self-confidence, more self-awareness, and more authenticity in the eyes of others, the more he can drive this social change.

If we are going to talk about a crisis of masculinity, then we have to see this crisis as an opportunity. An opportunity for change. Through the process of coming to terms with ourselves, we begin to ask questions and to define things in new ways, which, in turn, changes people's thinking, their attitudes, and their behavior. This process can be both frightening and unsettling, but it can also be liberating and exciting. Perhaps it is exactly this process that we can see happening all around us and that will eventually allow men to lead more authentic, intimate, emotional, and sensitive lives.

The clinical psychologist Martin Seager is one of the cofounders of the Male Psychology Network of British physicians and

psychologists, which organizes an annual conference on the subject
of men's mental health. Seager is convinced that the traditional rules
of masculinity put an enormous amount of pressure on men to
think, to feel, and to behave in a certain way. When I talked to him,
he summarized for me the rules of masculinity.

1. A real man is a fighter and a winner.
2. A real man is a provider and a protector (of women and
    children).
3. A real man is controlled and disciplined.

Seager doesn't believe that these social expectations will completely disappear, but he does have the impression that society is
currently in the process of changing and broadening the application
and the content of these rules. What does this process look like? Well,
providing for others could also mean providing for them at an emotional level, instead of just a financial and physical one. These are
all important and legitimate ways of being a provider. A man could
look after his partner by trying to be emotionally present and available. He could share childcare, which also represents a form of
masculine provision and masculine protection. If society as a whole
(and men themselves) expects men to fight and to win, then we
could also broaden our definition of what that means. What might
a contemporary form of masculine fighting look like in the twenty-
first century? How about fighting for something that matters to you
or fighting for a good cause? How about fighting for your family or
your relationship? And could success also mean having close and
emotionally satisfying relationships with other people, leading a
long psychologically and physically healthy life, and having a career
that gives your life meaning? If the only definition of success is status, if professional and sexual success only relates to material wealth,
then that can only lead to a situation in which most of us don't feel
successful and our attempts to become real men in our society are
going to falter and eventually fail.

To redefine these rules, however, men also need the support of women who allow them to be who they are. And they need the support of other men who treat them with warmth and acceptance and in doing so enable this emancipation from the narrow rules of masculinity.

SUMMARY

This is what the emancipation of men, which, to my mind, is long overdue, could look like. And what could it feel like? How about friendly, fatherly, brotherly, benevolent, accepting, equal, communal, generous, caring, and liberating? Both to ourselves and to others. Including instead of excluding. What would happen if men started to take more notice of their emotional needs and to verbalize them? If they showed the full spectrum of their feelings, not just anger and rage but also loneliness, sadness, helplessness, joy, and excitement? If our society was completely open to boys and men being emotional and sensitive and saw these qualities as something attractive and masculine? Just imagine if men were able to steadily free themselves from the strict categories of what is typically masculine and typically feminine and be less defined by them?

What would change in your friendships, in your relationships, in the way that you parent, in the career that you choose? The aim wouldn't be to become more feminine or to sweep aside any differences between men and women; that would be neither possible nor desirable. The aim would be to feel freer and lighter, to throw off that heavy old armor.

In order to achieve this, we need highly sensitive men who can be an example to others, showing less sensitive men that they can be sensitive, emotional, tactful, *and* masculine and that it's a great way to live your life. A few years ago, I had a long conversation with Christopher Germer, a clinical psychologist and the author of *The*

Mindful Path to Self-Compassion: Freeing Yourself from Destructive Thoughts and Emotions.[31] We covered many topics, including masculine identity, shame, introversion, and high sensitivity. We also spoke about how completely revolutionary it would be, and how much it would change the world, if every man started to try to deal with his feelings and could realize that everything that he felt, thought, and did was automatically manly because he was a man, whether or not society currently saw him as typically masculine. Germer hit the nail on the head when he summed up our conversation by saying, "A man is just a human being living in a male body. We sometimes forget that."

How can we all make sure that we remind ourselves of this more often?

John: "Free yourself from society's expectations."

I think John is a particularly good role model for highly sensitive men because as well as being a highly sensitive man, he is also a highly successful attorney in a professional field that we usually associate with traditional masculine attributes and behaviors. He also talks about how he has tried to free himself from society's expectation that a man should want to be sexually promiscuous. Interestingly, this is a subject that many highly sensitive men, whether gay or straight, have discussed with me.

When and how did you first notice you were highly sensitive?

That fact that I was more sensitive to stimuli than my peers began to crystalize when I was in my late teens. Looking back now, my first sense was that I couldn't "endure" activities that were typical for people my age, like going to parties and clubs, because I was too sensitive to noise. It wasn't until I was a student, around twenty-two, that I started to think that other people might feel the same way and I started to do some research and read around about it. That's when I came across the concept of high sensitivity.

What are the advantages and the disadvantages of being highly sensitive?

One man's meat is another man's poison, and high sensitivity seems to trigger specific characteristics that—depending on the situation—can be helpful or unhelpful. It means that you have an intense sensory perception, an intense life and experiences. But I could do without the intensity of experiencing acute overstimulation.

Looking back, what sort of messages or feedback would have been helpful to you?

In hindsight, I would've liked it if someone had explained to me why I was "different" and how I could deal with that. I would've found a role model really helpful, especially when I was going through puberty. Someone who got my sensitive disposition and could've helped me find my place in the world. Maybe it would've also been good if someone had more clearly communicated to me that it was "okay" to be how I am and that I don't need to achieve things to be recognized or loved even. On the other hand, the term *highly sensitive* wasn't around back then. And my father, who knew about my sensitive nerves, gave me some little practical tips that I still remember to this day. For instance, before my driving test, he instilled in me that I should take it all really slowly.

What are the particular challenges that highly sensitive men face in our society?

I feel like society sees sexually successful men as being promiscuous and also expects that men want to be promiscuous. Because of my high sensitivity, I don't find it easy to instigate cursory sexual contact. Not wanting to do it isn't an argument, though: a "real man" should want it. In this regard, I don't think that men have been successful at emancipating themselves completely from society's expectations.

How does your high sensitivity affect your relationships with other men?

This observation may be something that's just a coincidence, but I feel that I get along really well with gay men. Two of my good friends came out after I'd known them for a while. Other than that, I tend to be friends with women. I don't do very well with activities that are "typical for men." I have a particular problem with competitive sports, perhaps because I know that I don't have much of a chance in those sort of games. I am just better friends with women. My sense is that they are more communicative. I probably assume that men are going to be more shallow.

How does your high sensitivity affect your relationships with women?

I think that high sensitivity makes friendships with women easier. Depth of processing at an emotional level means that you can have deeper conversations. In relation to sexuality, I think I'm a bit insecure when it comes to recognizing sexual interest, eliciting it, and to attracting women. I think you need to exude a really robust self-confidence for that, which doubt-ridden highly sensitive men often don't have. In terms of romantic relationships, I lack a certain playfulness with women. But if I'm emotionally involved, it feels like the stakes are very high, because the threat of being deeply hurt is so high.

What are the advantages and the disadvantages of being highly sensitive at work?

I never felt like being highly sensitive played any kind of role in my professional life. Sometimes I'll be asked how a highly sensitive person deals with the sort of antagonistic situations thrown up by legal fights, which you experience a lot working as an attorney. But this is only an issue if you believe that the aggression in those situations is real and not just part of the game.

My advice for other highly sensitive men . . . ?
Free yourself from society's expectations about how you should behave, what your preferences should be, or how you define success or happiness. Accept that you're going to be following a different set of rules.

Understanding High Sensitivity: The Scientific Background and Why People Differ in Their Innate Sensitivity

Y OU MAY WELL HAVE READ a lot about high sensitivity in other books or online, thought long and hard about the term *high sensitivity*, and already decided that you're highly sensitive. Or perhaps you've read a couple of articles about high sensitivity, heard about it here and there, and wondered whether you, too, might be highly sensitive. Or perhaps you're not highly sensitive at all, but you have an inkling that your spouse, your partner, your son, your son-in-law, your brother, your father, or one of your friends might be highly sensitive and you want to better understand what it means. Maybe someone gave you this book as a present or lent it to you because that person thinks that you could be highly sensitive. Whatever the reason is that you're reading these pages, I'm really happy that you're here. Because the more people who know about high sensitivity and really understand what it is, the better.

In this chapter, so that you get a really clear idea of exactly what high sensitivity is, I want to give you a compact but detailed overview of the academic research on the subject. This will increase your knowledge about high sensitivity and give you a firm grounding in the theoretical background. I will also explain the scientific context, showing how high sensitivity complements the better-known term *introversion*. At the same time, it's important to me that you understand that the concept of high sensitivity is based on the results of numerous robust scientific studies from around the world and represents a serious field of scientific research. It is in no way some sort of "new age" phenomenon. One can get this impression when one sees the myriad ways in which people try to sell the term *high sensitivity* and the way it is sometimes presented in online forums. High sensitivity is neither a silver bullet nor some sort of sixth sense. Highly sensitive people haven't traveled from another galaxy, nor are they necessarily gifted. It is not a psychological disorder, but a neutral temperamental trait that can help to explain many things, but not all things. It is also very important to differentiate high sensitivity from a temporary psychological sensitivity during stressful life events or a short-term period of feeling thin-skinned after, for instance, suffering trauma or during a period of depression or anxiety. High sensitivity is not a temporary state, but a constant trait that you are born with and will carry with you for the whole of your life.

Sensitivity, Introversion, and Extroversion

We are all different, and we arrive in the world with some of these differences. Anyone who has kids or who has friends and family with kids knows that newborn babies already differ from each other, even in their very first few weeks of life. Before we have been influenced by experiences, other people, our education, or any number of other factors that help form our personalities, we are already reacting differently to stimuli and consequently display different behavioral tendencies. "She's a much worse sleeper than her sister," "She cries much more than her brothers and sisters," or "He feeds really slowly because he's always distracted by things he sees" are just a few of the kinds of comments I've heard from parents describing and comparing their children. So children's innate temperaments have a substantial influence on them and are observable from Day 1. And a child's temperament also has an influence on its parents' behavior, which, in turn, influences how secure the parent–child bond is. This means that differences in temperaments between parents and children can sometimes lead to problems in this relationship and that parents can sometimes become frustrated if they feel that their child has a "difficult" temperament. I can recall a highly sensitive client who was often yelled at and even punished by her stressed and overworked mother because, as a child, she cried far more often that her elder sister and her mother couldn't bear it.

If we are going to talk about temperament, this, of course, raises the question of what the term temperament actually means. The ancient Greek physician Hippocrates (c. 460–375 BC) was one of the first Western thinkers to tackle the question of temperament, developing his own temperamental theory. Since then, countless writers, philosophers, doctors, psychologists, and academics have explored the idea of temperaments and defined a range of different temperamental traits. To this day, research into human temperaments remains an important area of developmental psychology.

Professor Silvia Schneider of Ruhr University, Bochum, offers a clear and easily comprehensible definition of what temperament actually is: "The word temperament describes a constitutional factor that is inherited and which predisposes someone to react to situations and people in specific ways. Temperamental traits can be understood as those that form the basis for the development of the personality, appear early in life, are stable over time, and which are influenced by biological factors."[1]

Simply put, our temperament is the basis of our personalities and the complex interaction between our temperament and our environment forms our personality.[2] Researchers disagree on exactly how stable temperamental traits are. There is, nevertheless, broad agreement on the fact that our temperament represents a relatively permanent tendency that affects how we react and inter- act with the world from early childhood onward.

Carl Jung, the Swiss psychiatrist and psychoanalyst, was the first person to talk about "innate sensitivity." Jung believed that around 25 percent of all people are born with a particularly sensitive dispo- sition and that this sensitivity has a decisive influence on people's worldview. Jung introduced the terms *introversion* and *extroversion* into personality psychology to describe two different natures that influence people's perception, intuition, thinking, feelings, and be- havior. According to Jung, introverted people are more inclined to direct their energy and their attention inward and toward their inner processes (feeling and thinking, for instance), whereas extroverted people are more strongly inclined to direct their physical energy out- ward.[3] Since then, numerous researchers into personality traits, including Jung himself, have continued to develop the concept of introversion and extroversion.

One of these researchers was the German-born British psychol- ogist Hans Jürgen Eysenck, who related Jung's concept to Hippocrates's temperamental theory and believed that there is a neu- rological basis for the differences between introverted and extroverted people. In 1968, he described the typical introvert as someone who is quiet, introspective, rather reserved (except with very close friends), and loves books more than people. Introverts tend to make plans in advance, be cautious, and not like impulsive actions. They don't like arousal, approach daily life with a certain seriousness, and value a well-ordered life. Eysenck describes the typical extrovert as sociable, as someone who likes events, has many friends, needs people to talk to, and doesn't like being alone. Extroverts crave ex- citement, are constantly making the most of opportunities, react spontaneously, take risks, and are generally more impulsive.[4]

As such, Jung's concept of innate sensitivity began to shift to a difference between *observable* extroverted and introverted behaviors in people. Jung's theory of extroversion and introversion continues to be hugely important, and it has had a decisive influence on research into both temperament and personality. In the most commonly used model of personality psychology, the Big Five, extroversion is included alongside openness to experience, conscientiousness, agreeableness, and neuroticism. And there continues to be widespread interest in the concept of extroversion and introversion outside of academic research, as evidenced by the success of books like Susan Cain's brilliant bestseller, *Quiet: The Power of Introverts in a World That Can't Stop Talking*.

Another researcher influenced by Jung's theory of extroversion and introversion is Jerome Kagan, professor of developmental psychology at Harvard University. Based on the results of his longitudinal studies, begun in the 1970s, Kagan differentiates between two groups of children: *inhibited* children and *uninhibited* children. According to Kagan, these two types represent relatively stable temperamental traits that follow us throughout our lives and that can only be influenced by environmental factors to a limited extent. Schneider summarizes Kagan's results as follows:

> Behavioral inhibition can be defined as a withdrawn, cautious, avoidant, and shy behavior in new and unfamiliar situations, such as meeting new people or dealing with unfamiliar objects and environments. This behavior can already be evident at the age of eight months. In babies, behavioral inhibition manifests itself as an easily triggered irritability (for instance, crying or screaming), in infants as shy and anxious behavior, and in school children as socially withdrawn behavior. The stability of this temperamental trait into adolescence has been demonstrated in a number of studies.[5]

According to Kagan, around 20 percent of all children exhibit inhibited behavior. These children have a lower arousal threshold than other children, particularly in unfamiliar situations. This means that their sympathetic nervous systems respond in a more reactive way to these stimuli. The sympathetic nervous system is part of the autonomic nervous system, alongside the parasympathetic nervous system, which is involved in activities such as digestion when we are at rest. The sympathetic nervous system, on the other hand, is involved in stimulating activities that affect our heart rate, blood pressure, muscle tone, and metabolism. When confronted with an unfamiliar situation or a new stimulus, inhibited children—in contrast to uninhibited children—will exhibit shy, cautious, and withdrawn behavior, while simultaneously exhibiting increased stress symptoms in their sympathetic nervous system, such as muscle tension and a heightened heart rate.

Numerous other researchers on temperament, including the psychiatrists Alexander Thomas and Stella Chess, have developed a range of different categories and models to differentiate between various temperamental traits. In their longitudinal study on temperamental development, which ran from 1956 to the 1990s in New York, Thomas and Chess observed the behavioral characteristics of babies and defined nine new temperamental dimensions.[6] They were able to assign a clear temperamental type to 65 percent of the babies: 40 percent were categorized as "easy" babies, 10 percent were "difficult" babies, and around 15 percent were categorized as "slow to warm up." In a book on high sensitivity, you can probably guess that it is the babies who were "slow to warm up" that we are interested in. The babies in this group were withdrawn when they had to deal with new people or situations and needed more time to get used to them. This means that they were initially behaviorally inhibited, but they then particularly benefitted from repeated contact and increased familiarity with new situations, people, or objects.[7, 8] Their activity levels were lower and their sensitivity to subtle stimuli greater, and they reacted less emotionally than babies with "difficult" temperaments.

What these scientific findings suggest is that Jung was probably right when he posited that "many people are more sensitive than others from birth onwards." And it also seems to be the case that children described as "inhibited" have similar characteristics to those described in other studies as "slow to warm up": a stronger physical and emotional reaction to new and unfamiliar situations and stimuli and withdrawn behavior. What research has also been able to show is that alongside visible differences in behavior, there are also underlying physical and biochemical differences between inhibited and uninhibited children, as well as between extroverted and introverted adults. Introverted people, for instance, display a lower pain threshold and generally react more sensitively to external stimulation, such as visual and aural stimuli.[9] Both the British psychologist Jeffrey Alan Gray and the American psychiatrist C. Robert Cloninger have created influential models that suggest that personality differences between people can be explained by biological causes.[10]

For a long time, though, inhibited behavior among children had been judged negatively because it was connected with the development of anxiety disorders in adulthood. A sensitivity to new environmental stimuli was seen as representing a higher level of vulnerability or susceptibility and was thus judged to be a risk factor in the development of psychological problems, as well as being connected with shyness in both children and adults.

But could being more sensitive to external stimuli actually be advantageous? And could the same fundamental higher sensitivity be the underlying cause of all of these different behavioral characteristics, be they "slow to warm up," "behaviorally inhibited," "withdrawn," or "introverted"? It was these questions that a series of researchers began to ask in the 1990s, with fascinating results.

The Advantages of Being More Sensitive to Your Environment

So we have now learned that research into temperament suggests that, pretty much from birth onward, people register information from their environment differently from each other and also that they differ in their observable reactions and behaviors. These differences in sensitivity are not only seen among people, but have also been observed to date in over one hundred different animals, including rhesus monkeys, mice, dogs, zebra finches, fruit flies, and fish.[11]

Be it in a human being or a zebra finch, we can observe two distinct strategies when animals or people are faced with new or what initially appear to be threatening situations. One group behaves *reactively*, that is to say, they wait and become observant and cautious before they act. The other group, however, when faced with the same situation, reacts *proactively*, displaying daring and aggressive behavior and actively exploring the situation. Neither of these strategies is better than the other, both have advantages and disadvantages depending on the situation, so it seems that, for many species, it has paid off to retain both types.

Since the 1990s, a number of different models and hypotheses have been created to explain the individual differences in human sensitivity, including Jay Belsky and Michael Pluess's differential susceptibility theory, W. Thomas Boyce and Bruce J. Ellis's biological sensitivity to context, and Elaine Aron's sensory processing sensitivity. Although these theories all have their differences, the Swiss psychologist and researcher Pluess uses the umbrella term *environmental sensitivity* to broadly describe all of them.[12] What all of these theories have in common, in comparison to the earlier temperamental theories outlined above, is that they foreground the term *sensitivity*, which they judge neutrally, sometimes even identifying advantages associated with this higher sensitivity. Numerous studies over the past few years have clearly shown that those people who react more sensitively to their environment, react more strongly not only to *negative* events but also to *positive* events.

This means that being highly sensitive does not, as had previously been thought, necessarily lead to an increase in psychological vulnerabilities or disadvantages, but that, on the contrary, in the right surroundings, it can actually be an advantage. Both Belsky and

Pluess have been able to show that it is precisely those particularly sensitive children, whom we once called "slow to warm up," "difficult," or "behaviorally inhibited," who most profit from a caring and loving relationship with their parents and consequently receive better grades and display higher social competencies than those children with "easy" temperaments.[13] As Pluess said during a conversation with me, "We were able to show that children with 'difficult' temperaments developed better in positive, supportive surroundings than other children, precisely because their higher sensitivity meant that they reacted more strongly to positive influences." This is what Pluess calls "differential susceptibility"—that being sensitive means you suffer more from being in a negative environment, but also that you thrive more in a positive environment.

Belsky and Pluess believe that there are biological and evolutionary reasons why differences in individuals' sensitivities could be advantageous for a whole species when faced with uncertain conditions. If one strategy does not pay off, then the existence of the species could be assured by the alternative strategy. According to Belsky and Pluess, these differences manifest themselves in a more sensitive central nervous system and are influenced by genetics and prenatal and early postnatal factors. These individuals then react more sensitively to their environment and are thus more formed by it, a process that they can profit from.[14] It could thus be the case that differences in the sensitivity of people's nervous systems is a natural phenomenon.

Boyce and Ellis's theory of biological sensitivity to context is also based on the idea that being more sensitive is not necessarily a disadvantage for those affected, and can indeed be an advantage. But this is only the case when these particularly sensitive children grow up in a caring, loving, and supportive environment. Then the advantages of their sensitive nature becomes clear because they profit more strongly from these positive experiences and relationships than those who are less sensitive, precisely because they are so open to and affected by external influences and thus are more influenced by them than less sensitive children.

Boyce, who teaches at the University of California, Berkeley, has been able to observe that around 15 to 20 percent of all children react particularly sensitively to their environment. He refers to these children as "orchid children" and calls all other children "dandelion children," because, like robust dandelions, they can "grow anywhere" and have less "complicated care needs." The orchid children, on the other hand, are more pliable and react more sensitively to their environment. Boyce discovered that orchid children react particularly strongly to negative factors in their surroundings, which he measured based on their heart rates and their levels of cortisol (which is sometimes called the stress hormone because it is released at increasingly high levels when people are stressed). These children tended to react more often with behavioral problems when faced with negative situations in the family, such as money worries, illness, or parental conflict, in comparison with the dandelion children. In later life, these orchid children were more susceptible to developing problematic behaviors and psychological problems, including drug abuse and depression. But if those same particularly sensitive and malleable children grew up in low-stress, loving, and supportive surroundings, then they were happier, more productive, and healthier than the dandelion children.[15, 16]

What becomes clear when we take a close look at these recent studies is that all of us differ in our environmental sensitivity. And while particularly sensitive temperaments were described in earlier studies only indirectly and often negatively—with researchers believing that being more sensitive could make people more susceptible to psychological disorders—current research suggests that high levels of sensitivity are an essential and completely neutral trait. In other words, being more sensitive can be an advantage, but it can also be a disadvantage. This is completely dependent on which experiences the highly sensitive person has in the environment in which they grow up or live. The researchers whose work we have looked at in the second half of this chapter believe that natural selection led to the development of two discrete evolutionary strategies

that guaranteed the survival of our species. The advantage of the reactive or sensitive strategy could be that organisms, whether human
or animal, are more vigilant, sensitive, and adaptable when faced
with potential opportunities and threats in their environments and
social groups. Consequently, they are better able to adapt their future
behavior to these new situations.

So the next time that you as a highly sensitive man find yourself
in a full, loud, and sticky train car and feel unwell or tense while your
traveling companion appears to be calm, can concentrate on the
newspaper despite the noise, and is even able to order a hot coffee,
just remember that your sensitivity is not just a disadvantage, even
if it feels so in moments like this. Because it's likely that you're reacting more strongly not only to the negative aspects of this
situation but also to the positive: the golden field of flowers that the
train is speeding past, the colors of the sunset, the trees and the
shrubs, some good news in your friend's newspaper, or a funny or
loving interaction in the family sitting opposite you.

Elaine Aron's Concept of High Sensitivity

One of the researchers investigating sensitivity during the 1990s was
Elaine Aron, and she was the first to observe and identify the phenomenon of high sensitivity. Aron sees high sensitivity—or *sensory
processing sensitivity*, to use the scientific term—as a neutral, innate
temperamental trait. Highly sensitive people observe things in great
detail exhaustively, think longer and more deeply before they take
action, and generally react more emotionally to positive as well as
negative occurrences in their surroundings. This can be observed externally as a pattern of behavior in which people are more hesitant,
"slow to warm up," or "behaviorally inhibited." But Aron believes
that the underlying cause of this observable behavior is that highly
sensitive people process stimuli more deeply. Using the questionnaire that she developed during her research—the Highly Sensitive

Person Scale—Aron was able to show that highly sensitive people react more strongly to both positive and negative images, that they register small visual details more quickly, and even that they benefit more strongly from therapeutic interventions than non–highly sensitive people.[17, 18] Using brain imaging technology, Aron was able to show over the course of numerous studies that there were differences in the brain activity of highly sensitive and non–highly sensitive people. In highly sensitive adults, the areas of the brain connected with information processing, consciousness, empathy, and activity planning, such as the insular cortex and the inferior frontal gyrus, are all more active than in individuals who are not highly sensitive. The psychologist Bianca Acevedo summarizes the results of these studies as follows:

> Collectively, the present results support the notion that sensory processing sensitivity is a trait associated with enhanced awareness and responsiveness to others' moods, as it engages brain systems involved in sensory information processing and integration, action planning, and overall awareness. These findings highlight how the highly sensitive brain mediates greater attunement and action planning needed to respond to the environment, particularly in relevant social contexts.[19]

Aron's early research from the 1990s shows that around 15 to 20 percent of all people are highly sensitive, although Pluess suggests that the most recent research, in which Aron was also involved, estimates this figure to be around 30 percent. Pluess has also shown that there are three, rather than two distinct sensitivity groups, as previously thought, on a sensitivity continuum: a high sensitive group (31%), a medium sensitive group (40%) and a low sensitive group (29%). So not just "orchids" and "dandelions," but also "tulips."[20]

Aron differentiates high sensitivity from introversion and has been able to show that around 30 percent of all highly sensitive people are, in fact, extroverted.[21] This means, of course, that around 70 percent of all highly sensitive people are indeed introverted. Aron believes that high sensitivity can exist alongside a range of other apparently contradictory temperamental and personality traits, such as "sensation seeking."[22] The term *sensation seeking* was coined by the clinical psychologist Marvin Zuckermann, who has been researching this characteristic since the 1960s. He uses the term *sensation seeking* to describe people who seek out variety and new experiences, and, according to Zuckermann, it is a trait that is inheritable in 60 percent of cases.[23, 24] This characteristic tends to be connected to behaviors that can be described as "adventure-, risk- and excitement-seeking." Sensation seekers are more quickly bored than other people and thus seek out variety and potentially risky activities more often than other people. They tend to be restless when they find themselves in situations that offer little stimulation or variety. Zuckermann suggests that more men than women are sensation seekers and that those behaviors that accompany this trait tend to be moderated by age. Having a tendency to seek out risk, variety, and excitement, while also being highly sensitive, is something that Aron often compares to having "one foot on the brake, the other on the gas."[25]

Aron also differentiates between high sensitivity and neuroticism—the tendency to react anxiously or depressively. Aron believes that highly sensitive people only have a higher risk of developing anxiety, depression, or shyness in life if they had a childhood that involved significantly negative experiences and an environment that badly clashed with their temperaments. The particular malleability of highly sensitive children again plays a decisive role here, specifically the question of how well the attributes, expectations, behaviors, and challenges of a child's social environment fit their temperament—what in psychology we often call "goodness of fit." If the fit is good, or good enough, then, according to Aron, highly sensitive children will develop just as well, if not better, than children who are not highly sensitive, which tallies with the research of Boyce, Ellis, Belsky, and Pluess. It is, of course, completely possible that a highly sensitive adult will experience a depressive episode or other psychological problems in life, despite experiencing a safe and loving childhood, but what we can say is that high sensitivity *in itself* does not automatically lead to an increase in the likelihood of suffering from depression or anxiety.

SUMMARY

My hope is that you now feel that you have a broad enough knowledge about the academic background of high sensitivity and that you are better able to place the concept scientifically. Since the 1990s, high sensitivity, or sensory processing sensitivity, has represented a specific and active field of research that underpins the scientific basis of what Jung was already describing in 1913 as "innate sensitivity." Around the middle of the last century, this innate sensitivity was described using an array of different terms. High sensitivity has a biological and evolutionary explanation, can be demonstrated in measurable differences in brain activity, and has recently been connected to a range of genetic variations, including in the neurotransmitters (the messengers of our nervous system) serotonin and dopamine.[26, 27] For a long time, sensitivity was believed to be equivalent to introversion, despite the fact that we now know that high sensitivity and introversion are two separate things. These two phenomena do often go hand in hand, however, but we also know that around 30 percent of all highly sensitive people display extroverted behaviors in social settings. According to Aron, high sensitivity is a temperamental trait, whereas introversion and extroversion are personality styles that develop over the course of one's life and describe our social behavior. She thus believes that we are born highly sensitive, whereas introversion and extroversion are learned.

For the sake of our quality of life, our happiness, and our psychological health, it is very important that we are able to recognize whether we are highly sensitive or not. This is the question that we will be addressing in the next chapter, while tackling the typical characteristics and difficulties that highly sensitive men have to deal with in daily life.

Darryl: "For me, the positive aspects of my high sensitivity outweigh the negatives; the advantages and disadvantages are two sides of the same coin."

Darryl is in his early thirties. He is a musician and is training to be a masseur. His story illustrates how high sensitivity and the characteristics connected to it can be assets. He's found that aspects of his temperament are useful in his work as both a musician and masseur. And he actively seeks ways to accommodate his temperament; I like that he is seeking out other musicians to play with onstage rather than allowing his stage fright to force him offstage completely. In the interview, Daryl mentions a diagnosis of "social phobia," and it is important to mention here that there is a difference between high sensitivity and social phobia, because the latter is a psychological disorder, not a temperamental trait (see chapter 4). Social phobia is a distinct fear of being the center of attention in social situations and is accompanied by symptoms of anxiety, avoidant behavior, and distress. This is not necessarily the case with high sensitivity. Of course, it is possible for highly sensitive people to pick up and react more strongly to subtle social stimuli or develop social anxiety more rapidly in the face of negative social experiences than less sensitive individuals. It is also possible to be both highly sensitive and also socially anxious.

When and how did you first notice you were highly sensitive?
In 2008, my cognitive behavioral psychotherapist—who I was seeing about my social anxiety—pointed out that I might be highly sensitive. I believe that my high sensitivity contributed to the devel-

opment of my social anxiety, but only in interaction with some unpleasant external influences from my childhood. I then read a few
books about the subject and was immediately convinced that my
therapist was right, because I saw myself in so many of the highly
sensitive characteristics described, which I hadn't previously had any
explanation for and which didn't seem to be completely explained
by social phobia.

What are the advantages and the disadvantages of being highly sensitive?

For me, the positive aspects of my high sensitivity outweigh the
negatives; the advantages and disadvantages are two sides of the same
coin. The "advantages" for me are my rich inner life, my strong fantasies and creativity, my feel for aesthetic things, and the ability to be
on my own without feeling bored. I'd also say that I have a very clear
sense of justice, that I'm very empathetic, thorough, and conscientious.
The "disadvantages" are that I get quickly overstimulated, I'm a perfectionist, I tend to doubt myself and be very self-critical, and I'm
sometimes quite hesitant and not very spontaneous. It can also sometimes be a problem that I need time out, to protect myself from too
much stimulation, and that I often feel emotionally overwhelmed.

Looking back, what sort of messages or feedback would have been helpful to you?

"If you're different from other people, that doesn't mean that
there's something wrong with you; it means you're special."

"Always listen to what your body and your intuition are trying to
tell you and stick with that."

"Your sensitivity is really important for society as a whole. You
can do a lot of good."

"The particular way you see the world is an asset."

"Feelings are never right or wrong; (we can just deal with them
well or less well)."

"It's completely fine if you're shy, quiet, or withdrawn."

What are the particular challenges that highly sensitive men face in our society?

I think as a highly sensitive man I have traits that might be seen as "feminine" and other traits that would be seen as "masculine." Sometimes I'm quite reserved, quiet, and need harmony in my life. I think a lot about my emotional life, practice yoga and meditation, and am interested in spiritual things. I react sensitively to physical violence or shocking images in, for instance, films. I'm also not very interested in cars or technical things, and my physical build is quite slim. At the same time, I also have lots of "manly" characteristics and preferences, like football and drinking beer. I like to exhaust myself physically and can also be dominant and strong-willed. Generally, my sense is that many women, but also men, actually really value this mixture of "feminine" and "masculine" characteristics.

How does your high sensitivity affect your relationships with other men?

I have as many male friends as female friends and don't see many differences in those relationships. In terms of my relationships with men, it could be a disadvantage that I have a strong need for harmony, have difficulties setting boundaries, and am not interested in competition among men. However, one advantage in the way I relate to other men is that I often pick up on things that they don't notice about themselves, like particular feelings. For instance, my brother and my father—they both have a real flair for analytical thinking, but I would say that they find it hard to access their feelings, like anger or sadness. I feel like I'm sometimes able to help them by acting like a kind of "emotional mirror." At the same time, I do think I have to be really careful with them and make sure I'm "speaking their language," because I think I've been addressing my feelings in a far more direct way for a lot longer, including with two therapists. I've noticed that men who are comfortable with themselves and with their masculinity don't have any problems with my high sensitivity and, in fact, are able to value it. On the other hand, men who have problems with their self-worth, if, for instance, they don't acknowledge the shy or introverted sides of their personality, tend to demean highly sensitive characteristics in other men. I've experienced that myself regularly, also with women.

How does your high sensitivity affect your relationships with women?

I am often reserved and cautious when it comes to approaching new people and need a lot of time to open up. When it comes to talking to attractive women, to flirting and initiating intimacy, I'm often very hesitant and tense. In my experience, highly sensitive and shy men have a far harder time when it comes to all of that, because in our society it's sadly still the case that people expect men to make the first move, to "bowl women over," and to actively initiate sex. Because of that, I'm still quite unhappy with my sex life. But the moment that I've got past that first stage, then everything's great, and I'm sure that my high sensitivity plays a role in that. I can have very intense, deep conversations with women about feelings, about spiritual topics and about relationships, and I find it easy to put myself in my partner's shoes. I also experience sex with a woman very intensely.

What are the advantages and the disadvantages of being highly sensitive at work?

I recently started the training to become a masseur. My high sensitivity helps me to intuitively notice things about my clients. I'm very perceptive when I work and often need to process that, usually by taking a little break between clients. As a musician, my high sensitivity really helps my creative process: intuition, empathy, a feel for aesthetics and details, but also for the bigger picture, conscientiousness, and the ability to really immerse myself in my art. At the same time, my precision can also quickly turn into perfectionism. If I have to be the center of attention, have to present myself and sell myself (whether online or onstage), then I feel very inhibited and often get very nervous, especially if I have to stand on the stage on my own and sing. Because of this, I haven't performed very much, which has held me back professionally. I'm currently looking for other musicians to play with me to help me deal with that.

What's your advice for other highly sensitive men?

Unconditionally accept your own personality, your past, and your life story, as well as your present situation in life. Research your high sensitivity by reading books and talking to other people about it. I also think that positively reinterpreting life events from your past and your characteristics with your newfound knowledge about your high sensitivity is also really important. At the same time, you need to organize your own life according to your highly sensitive nature and stop trying to constantly fulfill everyone else's expectations. Pay more attention to the signals that your body's giving you and to your intuition, by practicing mindfulness meditation, for instance. And last but not least: take a walk in the woods—barefoot is best!

CHAPTER 3

Identifying High Sensitivity: Am I Highly Sensitive?

H OW DO I KNOW WHETHER I'm highly sensitive? And what are the implications of being born with a particularly sensitive and reactive central nervous system? These are the questions that we're going to deal with in this chapter. In the first two chapters, we looked at masculinity and the psychological health of modern men and talked about the urgent need to emancipate men from traditional models of masculinity, then we took a detailed look at the scientific research that underpins high sensitivity. This chapter aims to help you build up a clear picture of the ways in which high sensitivity can manifest itself in our everyday lives and whether you yourself are highly sensitive.

Am I a Highly Sensitive Man?

"I react strongly to criticism." "People are always telling me that I'm too sensitive." "I wish I had thicker skin." "I've been really sensitive ever since I was a child." "I get quickly stressed and find loud music and noisy surroundings hard to deal with." "I'm very emotional." "I'm always reflecting on things." These are just a few of the typical things I've heard from the highly sensitive clients that I've met over the past few years. Do any of these kinds of thoughts ring a bell with you? If so, this might be a sign that you are also highly sensitive. (Of course, these sorts of thoughts can also have a range of other causes and could, for instance, be the result of short-term psychological issues, in which case it's very important that you reflect on the broader context of your feelings, perhaps with a trained therapist.)

Often men come to my practice because they feel depressed or anxious or they are experiencing problems forming relationships with other people. It is thus often the case that we only begin to explore high sensitivity during the later stages of therapy, once the initial psychological issues have been addressed. And this was exactly what happened with the male client whom I mentioned at the beginning of the book who first alerted me to high sensitivity. There are also, of course, many highly sensitive men who are psychologically stable and do not require any kind of psychotherapy or who live harmoniously with their sensitivity. These men might never learn about their own high sensitivity.

So what are the signs of a highly sensitive temperament? A while back, I was sitting in a café with an old friend, whom we'll call Oliver, and we were chatting about high sensitivity. He listened attentively to what I was saying, thought about it, and then suddenly asked whether I thought that he could be highly sensitive. I had, in fact, for some time thought that Oliver was highly sensitive, but I hadn't talked to him about it because I felt it might be perceived as being presumptuous and I felt like it wasn't something that had particularly been bothering him. In fact, I thought that Oliver had long since learned to live in harmony with his high sensitivity, creating a lifestyle for himself that fitted well with his temperament. If we take Oliver as a case study, then what were the signs that he is highly sensitive that I picked up on?

Oliver

Oliver works freelance and really enjoys this way of working. A few years ago, he stopped freelancing and started working full time in a typical office environment, which was a big challenge for him. There were a number of reasons for this, including the fact that he found the noise level in the office and the constant conversations between colleagues very distracting and exhausting. He was not in full control of his workload anymore and was very aware of whether his boss and his colleagues were in a good mood or not. Oliver is someone who thinks a lot about things—about his life, about the lives of his friends, about politics and culture. Nowadays, Oliver works freelance, again in an office, but one that he shares with a single colleague. He finds life much easier than he did when he worked in a large office. Even in this new setup, however, when things get too loud, he wears earplugs so that he can concentrate. Outside of work, he is very sensitive to sounds, smells, and temperatures. For instance, he doesn't particularly like going to restaurants or bars that are too hot and quickly feels unwell when he has to. He is also very sensitive to perfumes.

Oliver very quickly notices visual details and changes in his surroundings. In a restaurant, he once commented that the light had a "hint of grey in it." He is emotional and was seen as the "sensitive one" in his family. He likes to make plans, loves structure, doesn't like surprises, and very rarely takes risks, which is sometimes a disadvantage when it comes to meeting potential girlfriends. In these situations, he often feels tense and nervous. When it comes to making a decision, he will research it very thoroughly. In other words, he is the very opposite of impulsive.

Oliver is sensible and thoughtful when it comes to structuring his own life and being in touch with other people. I find him to be very analytical, warm, and empathetic, and he has a good feel for other people. He likes to socialize, but he regularly needs time alone or to be somewhere quiet, spending a lot of time in the park near his apartment. He doesn't like multitasking, which quickly stresses him out. He is also overwhelmed by bustling environments, such as the subway. He is funny and enjoys life, appreciates things, and likes long conversations with friends, preferably somewhere cozy in a small group of people he knows, rather than in a large group. When he is in a large group of people, he first observes the group for a while before he'll start chatting. When he gets excited about something, like a present or a fun evening out, then he gets really excited and you can really sense his joy. All of these qualities make Oliver a great friend, and all of his friends, me included, appreciate him a lot.

This profile of Oliver helps us understand how the typical characteristics of a highly sensitive temperament are triggered in daily life and in contact with other people. It also illustrates how important it is that there is a good fit between our temperament and our environment. Of course, we must be careful about making generalizations, because there are also many differences between highly sensitive people, but there are also numerous recognizable similarities, tendencies, and typical patterns and reactions.

Elaine Aron describes four indicators that we can use to judge whether we are highly sensitive, which she refers to using the acronym DOES.[1]

1. **D**epth of processing
2. **O**verstimulation
3. **E**motional reactivity, including empathy
4. **S**ensitivity to subtle stimuli

According to Aron, all four factors need to be present in a person from childhood onward and cannot be a direct consequence of a psychological illness or the experience of trauma (for instance, sexual, physical, or emotional abuse or violence over a short or long period of time). This is important to note, because it helps us understand the difference between high sensitivity and psychological problems or trauma. Sometimes clients use high sensitivity to explain away serious psychiatric problems, despite the fact that they don't exhibit all four of Aron's DOES indicators. This is understandable, because high sensitivity is not a pathological condition and is thus arguably less stigmatizing and shame inducing than being diagnosed with a psychiatric disorder. But this mislabeling will not serve the person well; it is very important that the person in question receives suitable therapeutic treatment for that specific condition. It can, of course, also be the case that both situations occur simultaneously, as in a highly sensitive person who is experiencing a crisis or suffering from a psychological illness. But, as we have seen with Oliver, this does not have to be the case if we are able to find a good way of living in harmony with our temperament. Let's take a closer look at these indicators of high sensitivity so that we can get a clearer idea of exactly what they mean and how they manifest themselves.

Depth of Processing

Depth of processing is the key characteristic of high sensitivity, from which the other three indicators all stem. Depth of processing can't be observed externally, but can be witnessed indirectly in people who think deeply about things and experience strong feelings in response to their surroundings and the experiences that they have. It is a high sensitivity, a "delicacy" when faced with both positive and negative sensations and nuances in the world, and the deep way in which one deals with and processes what one has experienced. In brain scans of highly sensitive people, we can actually see stronger activity in the regions of the brain that deal with the perception of details and information.

What this means on a practical level is that you may, for instance, be someone who thinks a lot about spiritual and philosophical questions. It may mean that you find decisions difficult to make or often need more time to weigh things out. It may mean that you like to think analytically and that you find it easy to think abstractly and laterally about problems. It may mean that you appreciate and seek out depth. It may mean that you feel the suffering of other people and animals so strongly that it is almost as if the things you've witnessed happening to them have happened to yourself. This means that you tend to react with empathy, because you find it easy to sympathize with other people's feelings. Depth of processing can also exhibit itself in the way that highly sensitive people sometimes need more time before they start speaking or acting. They reflect often on the past and the future. Their lack of immediate response should not be mistaken for disinterest or indifference. They are usually anything but numb and indifferent. They are usually awake, sympathetic, observant, and engaged with themselves and with whatever or whoever they're facing—be it people, experiences, art, literature, or films.

Everything that they experience, they process deeply, and every experience leaves behind traces in the form of thoughts, feelings, impressions, bodily sensations, memories, and fantasies. Much more so than in people who react less sensitively to their environment. It is as if the mind and the body of a highly sensitive person are a seismograph that is able to pick up subtle vibrations in the ground, responding far more quickly and reacting far more strongly. Sometimes this can be pleasant, because it can be an enriching experience that makes life vital and varied. But sometimes it can be tiring and stressful, making you feel like you just want to notice, perceive, think, and feel less. When the things you experience are processed very deeply, then this is true of all experiences that you have in life, whether negative or positive. (You'll recall in the last chapter that we talked about the idea that highly sensitive people profit from positive experiences more than less sensitive people, but that they also react more strongly when faced with negative experiences, exhibiting problem behavior, anxiety, and depression. This is called the differential susceptibility theory.)

Let's think about Oliver again. Which of his characteristics or behaviors would we assign to depth of processing?

- A feel for other people's moods and a strong reaction to them in that they elicit lots of thoughts and feelings in him.
- The tendency to reflect and think deeply, being emotionally and cognitively engaged with the experiences he has.
- Making decisions conscientiously. Deeply and intensely weighing pros and cons before making a decision.
- Having the ability to put himself in other people's shoes, but also enjoying analytical thinking.
- Appreciating and taking part in deep, serious discussions and conversations with friends and partners.

And here are a few other characteristics and behaviors that suggest depth of processing that I've noticed among highly sensitive clients of mine:

- The tendency to know oneself fairly well, often based on the fact that highly sensitive people think a lot about things, including themselves.
- The ability to quickly learn from past experiences and then adapt one's behavior in the future.
- Reacting intellectually and emotionally to experiences in the past more strongly than other people.
- Quickly finding superficial conversations and small talk stressful, tiring, or boring.
- Occasionally thinking that it would be nice not to "have to constantly think about everything all the time," while also appreciating depth and seeking it out in conversations with others.
- The ability to see circumstances from many different perspectives.
- Being disposed to "perfectionism," in the sense that one works very thoroughly, deals with things very conscientiously, and thinks a lot about what one does. (This can also, of course, be a dysfunctional, overcompensatory

strategy in people with low self-worth who are trying to be particularly perfect.)

- The ability to clearly remember past events, often because the experience is invested with a high level of emotion.
- A tendency to fantasize, to daydream, to conjure up a lot of mental images, to be creative.
- Quickly becoming tired and overwhelmed when one has to multitask.
- The urge to take short breaks between activities, often because one has been so involved in an activity and needs a moment to regroup.
- Jumpiness, because one is so deeply in thought or involved in something that one didn't immediately spot the new stimuli. "Being lost in one's thoughts," describes this phenomenon well.

Overstimulation

If you react particularly sensitively to your environment and you deeply process the information and stimulation around you by observing, reflecting, feeling, and reacting, then this overstimulation can quickly lead to a feeling of overarousal. All people inevitably reach a high level of arousal if they experience a very high pitch of stimulation. In 1908, psychologists Robert M. Yerkes and John Dillingham Dodson introduced the Yerkes-Dodson law, which stated that people are most productive when they experience a medium level of arousal, not a very high or a very low level.[2] Essentially, our arousal level represents the level at which our nervous system is being activated. When we react to external and internal stimuli and process them, our physiological arousal increases, which, in turn, influences our feelings and thoughts. When this arousal level is too high, our well-being and our cognitive abilities begin to drop, which can manifest itself in difficulties concentrating, struggling to come up with ideas, and blanking (the dreaded situation in which one completely forgets what one has learned and is unable to perform as usual). We also experience a high degree of physical and emotional tension, sometimes even anxiety. This high degree of tension is often accompanied by a raised heart rate, shallow breathing, hot and flushed, increased sweating, and the need to urinate; in other words, our sympathetic nervous system is going into overdrive.

Under these circumstances, we often automatically and unconsciously attempt to bring our level of arousal back to the medium, optimal range. After a difficult and long day in a busy office, for instance, we might seek out the quiet of a garden or a park, or when we feel bored we might seek out friends or participate in some sport or activity. In both cases, what we're attempting to do, often unconsciously, is to regulate our level of arousal.

Because of their very reactive and sensitive central nervous systems, highly sensitive people process information very deeply and as such become overaroused and overstimulated far more quickly than people who are less sensitive to their environment. When this happens, this overstimulation can manifest itself as a feeling of physical or emotional tension, which is often perceived as agitation, nervousness, or unease. Often, highly sensitive people will describe overstimulation as just "stress" or "irritability," and it is usually the biggest challenge that their high sensitivity poses. This is likely because most highly sensitive people experience this overstimulation on a daily basis and it is often very hard to avoid these situations. A busy supermarket, a full restaurant with loud music, a long meeting at work, a presentation in front of a lot of people, a lively children's birthday party, or a noisy open-plan office—all of these are typical locations and situations full of sensations and stimuli that need to be processed.

A brief spell of overstimulation can be unpleasant but is not dangerous, whereas chronic overstimulation, underpinned by a high level of cortisol, can have negative consequences for our physical and mental health. In order to prepare our body to deal with stress-ful situations—fight or flight—our adrenal medulla pumps out the hormone adrenalin. If we are stressed over an extended period, the cortisol levels in our blood rise. Research has recently shown that having chronically high levels of cortisol can lead to interrupted sleep patterns, irritability, anxiety, high blood pressure, digestive problems, exhaustion, and depression.[3] It is therefore particularly important that highly sensitive people find a way of avoiding over-arousal caused by too much stimulation, take regular breaks, and generally try to lead a life in which they are not in a permanent state of overstimulation.

It's important to say at this point that this state of overstimula-tion should not be confused with symptoms of hypervigilance brought on by trauma, such as problems sleeping, jumpiness, and increased irritability. Aron sees overstimulation as one of the four central indicators of high sensitivity, which is based on being born with a sensitive nervous system and not with a trauma that one has experienced in life.

A male client of mine compared the feeling of overstimulation as "being full"—as if one can't absorb anything else because one is "full up" with so much information, stimuli, and the weight of processing these things emotionally and cognitively. A feeling that one might "burst" if one has to remain in that state of overstimulation. Another client described his experience of overstimulation as follows:

> When I feel overstimulated—and that happens quite often—then I always have the feeling that my perception shifts slightly. It's as if everything around me becomes a little sharper, louder, or more precise, before I feel this re-ally strong desire to retreat and recover, because I feel so exhausted afterwards. Typical situations that trigger this are dinners with lots of colleagues, or even friends, team meetings, but also when I'm alone and trying to concen-trate on work and my kids are being noisy in the next

room or the radio is on. I can't deal with those kinds of situations for very long, because I quickly feel really tense and unwell.

This client is describing something very typical for highly sensitive people: after a situation or a period of overstimulation, you feel a strong desire to retreat to somewhere quiet, preferably a calm room, in order to recover from the situation, to lower your sense of being overstimulated, and to digest what you have just experienced. This might be a quiet room in your home; it might mean going outside or just finding the quietest corner of the party. Once your arousal level has dropped back down to a medium level, a feeling of well-being returns along with a sense of inner calm. If your arousal level drops too low, however, you experience a sense of boredom. Highly sensitive people experience boredom less often than less sensitive people because they are inclined to higher rather than lower levels of arousal. Everyone, whether highly sensitive or not, wants to maintain an optimal level of arousal and avoid feeling bad when they are over- or understimulated. But for highly sensitive people, the depth with which they process stimuli from the world around them and their internal processes means that they become overstimulated much more quickly.

Let's think about Oliver again. Which of his characteristics or behaviors would we think of as being evidence of *overstimulation*?

- The feeling that highly stimulating places make him more tense, more nervous, more restless, more agitated, and more stressed. These feelings are often accompanied by cognitive and physical symptoms, such as shallow breathing, sweating, muscle tension, feeling hot, and trouble concentrating.
- A preference for structure, repetition, planning, and routine, rather than spontaneity and wanting to constantly experience new stimuli and new sensations. A sense that

unfamiliar situations with lots of new stimuli can quickly
make him feel overstimulated.
- A feeling of nervousness, agitation, physical discomfort, or
tension in some social situations that are perceived as
being overstimulating. This is based less on feelings of social anxiety about being judged negatively by others, as is
the case with people who are socially phobic, and far more
about the absorption and processing of many internal and
external stimuli and new sensations.

Ever since I started working with highly sensitive clients, I have
also noticed the following characteristics and behaviors connected
with overstimulation:

- A tendency to come to terms quite slowly with big life
changes: things such as moving, changing jobs, going off
to a university, becoming a parent, having children leave
home, retiring, and sometimes even reaching the end of
holidays and the beginning of the work week.
- A tendency to disparage oneself when one feels overstimulated. ("Why can't I just relax?" "Everyone else is dealing
with the situation so much better than I am," "Everyone's
noticed how tense and agitated I am," "Something's wrong
with me," "Oh, here it goes again," etc.)
- The desire to "feel calmer inside" being a constant theme
in one's life.

Emotional Reactivity (Including Empathy)

The third indicator of high sensitivity is a generally high emotionality, which is not limited to certain situations or specific feelings and
which often accompanies a depth of processing and overstimulation.
It is important to note here that this again relates to both positive

and negative feelings and is not related to very specific situations in which these feelings relate to a person's negative life experiences. In other words, a tendency to react to things more emotionally than others do in similar situations and to do so whether such things are pleasant or unpleasant and in whichever situation they take place. This emotional reactivity must have been observable since childhood (you'll recall the behaviorally inhibited children mentioned in the last chapter who at just a few months old reacted more emotionally than other children to unfamiliar situations and toys) and must not be the consequence of a traumatic experience. This differentiation is important, because the feeling of numbness that can follow a traumatic event for anyone can also entail feelings of anxiety and depression. But when we're talking about emotional intensity in the context of high sensitivity, we're talking about the broad spectrum of *all* human feelings.

Highly sensitive people are more affected by things that they experience and react more emotionally to them, whether it's joy and gratitude following a party with good friends, the disappointment of failing an exam, or dealing with criticism. All feelings are perceived more strongly, which brings a range of benefits but also numerous challenges. To add to this, feelings are always accompanied by thoughts, physical sensations, memories, images, and fantasies. Also typical for highly sensitive people, and connected to emotional reactivity, is a high capacity for empathy, supported by findings that show that the area of the brain containing "mirror neurons" is more activated in highly sensitive people. Mirror neurons are nerve cells in our brain. When we witness something, these neurons exhibit a pattern of activity that corresponds to the pattern that would have been activated if the same thing had happened to us. As such, they create the neurological foundation for us to empathize with other creatures. Empathy can be understood as "the ability to sympathetically understand the interior lives of other people, including their emotions, thoughts, needs, and motives."[4] Highly sensitive people are therefore usually very good at putting themselves in other people's shoes. What does the person opposite me think and feel? What is important to them? What are their needs? And what do the expressions of the other person, their words, their phrases, their thoughts trigger in me? These are the sort of automatic processes that one would categorize as empathetic processes.

What effect does being highly empathetic have in our daily lives? Highly sensitive people often tell me that they do a lot of volunteer work or that they're vegetarian or vegan. They are often very moved when they see homeless people on the street or starving children on television, and they reflect on these images for a long time (a good example of the ways in which *depth of processing* and *emotional reactivity* often operate in tandem). Friends and family will often think of them as "warm, always ready to help, and sympathetic." Many such people go through periods in which they can't watch any news or don't want to read the newspaper because they have the feeling that this concentration of suffering is too much for them.

At this point, it is also worth reminding ourselves that all highly sensitive people are different. It may be the case, for instance, that a highly sensitive man has a lot of empathy for factory-farmed animals and has therefore become a vegetarian or vegan, whereas another highly sensitive man might have a huge amount of sympathy for children and old people, but be less concerned about animals.

If we return to my friend Oliver, which behaviors and characteristics did he describe that we might think of as representing *emotional reactivity*?

- Reacting with strong emotions to pleasant stimuli and situations, such as birthdays, celebrations, or good conversations with friends, but also to unpleasant stimuli, such as his boss being in a bad mood or being in a loud office with difficult colleagues.
- A good intuition for other people and the ability to quickly perceive how they feel or whether they need something to make them feel better.

- Often described by his friends as warm, empathetic, and loyal.

I have also often noticed the following traits in my highly sensitive clients:

- They are quickly moved to tears when watching a sad film or reading a moving book.
- They are very affected by violent scenes in films or on the news.
- They experience intensively emotional reactions, even when they generally feel content and emotionally stable in their lives.
- They experience stronger pleasant and unpleasant feelings in situations that don't affect other people as much. This could be feeling very nervous on their first day in a new job, before giving a public presentation, or on a first date. But this is also true of positive feelings, such as joy when an old friend calls or when they're looking forward to their next holiday.
- A strong emotional reaction to criticism—often in the form of shame, a sense of being inferior, self-doubt, or anger.

Sensitivity to Subtle Stimuli

What do we mean exactly when we talk about sensitivity to subtle stimuli, and what are some of the concrete examples of this phenomenon? The first thing that comes to mind for me is a client who told me about her routine of changing her bedsheets once a week because after just a few days her bedding began to feel unpleasant on her skin. Another client of mine never wore socks or any kind of clothing that contained nylon or polyester because he immediately felt "too hot and unwell." He also sometimes had trouble sleeping in his apartment because of the noise coming from the street, although his girlfriend at the time hadn't even noticed the noise. After he'd pointed it out, she remained unbothered by it. Another client used to cut the labels out of his clothes because he found it "unpleasant" to have them next to his skin.

In all of these cases, it is not in, fact, the sensory organ in question that is better developed, but rather the deeper processing of the stimuli that is the marker of high sensitivity. In other words, highly sensitive people don't hear or see better than other people, but what they do perceive is processed more deeply and resonates in them longer. According to Aron, "Sometimes sensory sensitivity manifests as a low threshold, sometimes as the ability to distinguish subtleties, and sometimes as low tolerance of high levels of sensory input. Often all three are present."[5]

When I was working at the psychiatric hospital in London, the open-plan office shared by the therapists was in the basement. The room only had a few windows and was very dark. The room was lit by bright fluorescent strip lighting, and it was very noticeable that the fifteen therapists who worked there quickly split into two groups. One group didn't think the lighting was great, but they weren't that bothered about it and they rarely noticed it during the day. The other group found the lighting terrible and very unpleasant and could never get used to it. This group of therapists developed a range of sometimes very creative ideas to alter the lighting in their little pockets of the office and create a more pleasant atmosphere. This always struck me as a good example of the ways in which different people can react completely differently to the same stimulus (in this case, the fluorescent lighting), and I appreciated that, in the office, certain people processed this stimulus more deeply than others. This manifested itself in their sensitivity threshold and their limited tolerance to the stimulus.

Our sensitive, physiological perception of the world through our sensory organs can be related to hearing, seeing, smelling, tasting, and touching, and also to our perception of pain and of temperature.

I have often observed that it's very typical that highly sensitive people often have a marked aversion to extremes of temperature, whether hot or cold; that they often find loud, full, or busy places quickly overstimulating and thus prefer surroundings without lots of stimuli, be it a calm room, an empty museum, or a quiet garden; and that they are often very sensitive to smells and sounds, having to turn off music, for instance, if they need to focus on work. Many highly sensitive people have also told me that they react particularly strongly to coffee, alcohol, and medication; that they quickly feel aggravated when they're hungry; and that they quickly notice subtle changes in their environment, like a piece of furniture that's been moved, a friend's new haircut or glasses, or a new picture or a newly painted wall in someone's home. Wearing uncomfortable shoes or tight clothes, or even scratchy or rough materials, is, of course, unpleasant for most people, but it is certainly the case that some people find it much more unpleasant than others.

What are the signs of *sensitivity to subtle stimuli* in Oliver's behavior?

- The ability to quickly perceive subtle visual details and changes.
- A high sensitivity to smells, noises, and temperatures.
- Quickly feeling tense and unwell in places that overstimulate his senses, such as loud and full offices, hot restaurants with bright lighting, and busy trains on the metro.

Over the past few years, I've also been able to notice a few other common traits in highly sensitive clients that we might connect to sensitivity to subtle stimuli.

- Reacting strongly to other people's voices, particularly when they're perceived as being too loud or too shrill.
- The perception of subtle social signals in interactions with other people that others often don't notice. This can become challenging in common social situations, such as

meetings at work, group settings at school or university, or dinner with friends, because highly sensitive people are often able to "read between the lines" and perceive many subtle social stimuli.

- A strong connection to nature. Often highly sensitive people feel that they are most able to relax when they're outside, whether that's in the woods, in or on the water, in a garden, or walking through fields.
- Quickly getting quite stressed and overstimulated in busy surroundings, like a crowded street or market in a big city, when all of one's sensory organs are being stimulated at the same time.
- The sense that one is strongly affected by music, art, literature, and film, but also tactile stimuli, such as massage, swimming in water, or the feeling of sun on one's skin.

A Few Notes on DOES

I think it's important to again reiterate here that each of these four indicators (depth of processing, overstimulation, emotional reactivity, and sensitivity to subtle stimuli) must be present for someone to be considered highly sensitive, based on Aron's definition. At the same time, there are, of course, big differences among highly sensitive people in how these indicators manifest themselves and how regularly they occur, and the lists of examples above are certainly not exhaustive. Not every highly sensitive person, for instance, is sensitive to smells, and individual traits can manifest themselves to different degrees and be triggered differently in different situations. It is completely possible that a highly sensitive man who grew up with lots of siblings in a family where there were often lots of visitors is more used to a higher noise level and thus, as an adult, generally finds it easier to deal with similar social settings, compared with an only child who grew up in a very quiet household.

Alongside differences in our experiences and formative histories, how we're feeling on a given day, our mood, our age, and the context of a given situation all play important roles in how we feel and react. If on the whole we are experiencing relatively little stress and over-stimulation in our life at a given moment and are feeling pretty relaxed, then it's likely that we'd find it much easier to deal with short-term overstimulation, such as going to a party, than would be the case if we already felt chronically overstimulated and exhausted.

There are a whole range of factors that can affect the way our high sensitivity is experienced. Am I going into this potentially over-stimulating situation because it's important to me, or do I feel like I have to go? In other words, what is my motivation in this particular situation? Am I alone in this situation, or will there be other people there with me? Am I with my family, my partner, or my friends in an overstimulating situation, or am I surrounded by strangers who, per-haps, I don't like very much? Do I have good memories about the activity I'm doing or the place I'm doing it in?

All of these things help shape and influence the situation in question and can lead to differences in how highly sensitive people react. And we don't necessarily have to react to a given situation in exactly the same way as we reacted last time. Nevertheless, all four of the DOES indicators do need to be clearly recognizable and reg-ularly manifest themselves as a tendency in our lives for us to be considered highly sensitive.

It is also worth noting that not all four of these indicators will necessarily be felt as challenging or problematic as each other. A highly sensitive man like Oliver who works alone with one colleague in a quiet office is unlikely to see his sensitivity to subtle stimuli as something that's very problematic at work, compared with a highly sensitive man who has to work in a noisy environment in an open-plan office. A highly sensitive man who lives in a laid-back, rural setting is unlikely to feel overstimulated and consequently as over-aroused as someone who lives on a loud or bustling street in a busy city. It also possible that someone might find it easy to deal with sensitivity to subtle stimuli by always wearing particular materials or finding a quiet corner in the office to work at, but might really struggle with strong emotions when it comes to friends or relationships. In other words, not all of the DOES indicators have to have the same significance in your life, and certain indicators can be perceived more strongly in different phases of your life than in others.

The HSP Scale

As part of her research into high sensitivity, Aron developed a questionnaire consisting of twenty-seven questions: the Highly Sensitive Person Scale, better known as the HSP Scale. The questionnaire is a scientific measure, with a high degree of reliability, and it is regularly used in scientific research. Aron used her HSP scale to create a simple test that people can take themselves to help them work out whether they are highly sensitive or not. You often find versions of this test online. Aron is keen to point out that this single test should not be used alone to decide whether one is highly sensitive or not. The test should instead be used in combination with an in-depth exploration of one's own life story and the presence of the four DOES indicators mentioned above. At the same time, the statements that make up this test are very useful in helping us understand how high sensitivity often manifests itself in our everyday lives.

Instructions: Answer each question according to the way you personally feel. Check the box if the statement is at least somewhat true for you; leave it unchecked if the statement is not very true or not at all true for you.

- ☐ I am easily overwhelmed by strong sensory input.
- ☐ I seem to be aware of subtleties in my environment.
- ☐ Other people's moods affect me.
- ☐ I tend to be very sensitive to pain.

☐ I find myself needing to withdraw during busy days, into bed or into a darkened room or any place where I can have some privacy and relief from stimulation.

☐ I am particularly sensitive to the effects of caffeine.

☐ I am easily overwhelmed by things like bright lights, strong smells, coarse fabrics, or sirens close by.

☐ I have a rich, complex inner life.

☐ I am made uncomfortable by loud noises.

☐ I am deeply moved by the arts or music.

☐ My nervous system sometimes feels so frazzled that I just have to go off by myself.

☐ I am conscientious.

☐ I startle easily.

☐ I get rattled when I have a lot to do in a short amount of time.

☐ When people are uncomfortable in a physical environment, I tend to know what needs to be done to make them more comfortable (like changing the lighting or the seating).

☐ I am annoyed when people try to get me to do too many things at once.

☐ I try hard to avoid making mistakes or forgetting things.

☐ I make a point to avoid violent movies and TV shows.

☐ I become unpleasantly aroused when a lot is going on around me.

☐ Being very hungry creates a strong reaction in me, disrupting my concentration or mood.

☐ Changes in my life shake me up.

☐ I notice and enjoy delicate or fine scents, tastes, sounds, and works of art.

☐ I find it unpleasant to have a lot going on at once.

☐ I make it a high priority to arrange my life to avoid upsetting or overwhelming situations.

☐ I am bothered by intense stimuli, like loud noises or chaotic scenes.

☐ When I must compete or be observed while performing a task, I become so nervous or shaky that I do much worse than I would otherwise.

☐ When I was a child, my parents or teachers seemed to see me as sensitive or shy.

Analysis: According to Aron, it is very likely that you are highly sensitive if you ticked more than fourteen of these statements as "applicable." Although women are no more likely to be highly sensitive than men, women do tend to get higher scores on the HSP Scale. Her explanation for this reflects the gender-specific ideals in Western culture and the impression that men are less willing to admit that they are particularly emotional, sensitive, or quickly moved to tears.

Peter: "Try to accept the unique qualities of your temperament and begin to see the advantages."

Peter is in his mid thirties and is a psychology student. What I particularly like about his story is that the positives of his high sensitivity have prevailed, despite his problems with self-worth and shame. He talks about the kinds of women he is usually interested in and mentions that he often feels attracted to emotionally unstable women. This dynamic of highly sensitive people picking emotionally unstable partners is an interesting one and has come up a lot in my work. I suspect that the highly sensitive person who values emotional depth in everyday life is initially attracted to the depth and emotional intensity of these kinds of people.

When and how did you first notice you were highly sensitive?
During my childhood I was generally a pretty quiet and introverted child, preferring to wander around by myself at school

between classes or sit alone in the library reading magazines. I know that this behavior was considered "odd and different" by my peers. Although I have become much more extroverted and socially competent since my mid twenties, the underlying feeling has stayed the same. I'm still not comfortable in highly stimulating social environments, like parties or clubs, and I do need regular downtime and time to recover afterwards. Last year I stumbled upon Elaine Aron's book *The Highly Sensitive Person*, and it suddenly all made sense to me, and I understood why I'm so introverted and sensitive to subtleties. For a long time, I have struggled with low self-esteem, the feeling of not fitting in, the sense of not being able to change some of the things described above, but now I feel almost relieved because I know what the reason is. So the feeling of being highly sensitive has always been there, but I have only known about the term for about a year.

What are the advantages and the disadvantages of being highly sensitive?

I have noticed that most of my relationships are deep and emotional, which can be both stimulating and overstimulating. Mostly, I see this as positive. I also think that my sensitivity has helped me to disclose my thoughts and feelings to other people, which is a strength in close relationships and helps me to form them. In my opinion, being deep and reflective also benefits society as a whole as many important (and good!) decisions require deep reflection, and not a quick fix. I also really like that I see so much beauty in the world and feel touched by it: an emotional song, a happy face, or a bright painting.

I think that there are also some disadvantages to being highly sensitive that are mainly related to a society that emphasizes performance, flexibility, and the ability to do many things at once. I think highly sensitive men become overstimulated and stressed more quickly in the face of these requirements.

What are the particular difficulties of being a highly sensitive man in our society?

I think highly sensitive men suffer a lot more for not being socially dominant and extroverted in social situations, which society still expects from men. Personally, I experienced a lot of bullying during my adolescence because I was so sensitive and did not live up to the "male ideal."

What I also find difficult is when I feel anxious, stressed, or overstimulated, but others expect me to handle the situation in a calm and collected manner because I'm a man. I also avoid certain highly stimulating activities, such as skiing, climbing, or playing football, as I prefer more tranquil activities such as reading, reflecting, or walking in nature. I am much more a thinker than a doer! However, I often feel ashamed when I avoid these stimulating activities as I "should" be doing them. I also feel shame when I'm socially not as dominant as other men.

How does high sensitivity impact on your relationships with other men?

I am convinced that, generally speaking, my sensitivity has a positive impact on other men, but it depends on the situation. For example, when I meet a friend on my own or in a small group, I believe that they are often calm and comfortable in my company and feel able to disclose or share their problems. I know that many of my male friends see me as a deep and caring friend who they can talk intimately with. I think I influence them to reflect and think more deeply and to share their emotions more. However, a lot of men are not comfortable with deep conversations and a focus on thoughts and feelings. Certain situations require a more "shallow" conversational style or small talk, which I'm not very good at. I think some men get annoyed with me for not being good at small talk, and a couple of male friends have even ended their friendships with me because of my inability to "keep things light."

How does high sensitivity impact on your relationships with women?

When it comes to approaching women, I did have problems with self-esteem for most of my life. Having said that, I think that many women are quite reserved with men, but actually feel comfortable and relaxed in my company. My theory is that women tend to recognize empathy in others better than men do and find it appealing and calming. My tendency to disclose my thoughts and feelings to others appeals to many women, but I also think it can sometime become stressful and "a little too close" for them. Something else that I've realized is that I have a tendency to attract women who are emotionally unstable, in particular those who suffer from borderline personality disorder. I think this is because of my strong ability to show empathy and care, which is appealing to these women, and their need to be cared for is appealing to me. I think I have to be careful not to become codependent in these potentially dysfunctional relationships.

What are the advantages and the disadvantages of being highly sensitive at work?

I try to avoid jobs that focus relentlessly on flexibility and performance or that involve too much time pressure and multitasking. I think, as a highly sensitive man, I work best in a role in which I'm working with other people, because I have good people skills. I'm a loyal colleague, I take care of others, I'm reflective and can come up with good, creative ideas.

What are your priorities, and what lifestyle changes have you made?

I try to avoid highly stimulating environments and situations and always try to focus on one task at a time. I prioritize rest, sleep, and recovery above all, and try to engage in long-term projects that are meaningful to me and require reflection. I also try to avoid superficiality and unhealthy relationships.

Studying psychology, I prefer reading and reflection tasks as part of my studies. I always had problems with exams as I struggle with the time pressure. When I'm reading, I prefer a quiet place over a busy area with lots of other students. Sometimes group work can be good, but only if the group is small, reflective, and everyone is allowed to have their own opinions. Unfortunately, this is often not the case. When I'm reading, I usually take notes and take time to reflect on the content.

What's your advice for other highly sensitive men?

Try to accept your trait and start seeing the benefits of it. Seek quiet, secure, and predictable environments. Prioritize sleep, rest, and recovery. Enjoy thinking deeply about subjects and forming deep, meaningful relationships with others. But maybe most importantly, it's okay to be deep and a bit serious! You don't need to be shallow, even if society tells you differently.

CHAPTER 4

Everyday Effects of High Sensitivity and How It Differs from Psychological Disorders

I N THIS CHAPTER, WE'RE GOING to look at the particular challenges that many highly sensitive men are confronted with in their daily lives and learn why acceptance is the first step toward change. We are also going to address the differences between high sensitivity and psychological problems. This chapter also represents the final part of the theory section of this book and the transition into the practical section, which is going to introduce you to numerous strategies for dealing with your high sensitivity in a much better way.

OK, I'm Highly Sensitive—What Now?

I hope that at this point in the book you feel that you have a really solid understanding of what high sensitivity is, what the scientific explanations behind it are, and what the four DOES indicators of a

particularly sensitive temperament are. If at this point you think that
you are a highly sensitive man, then we need to take a look at what
consequences that might have for your everyday life and what the
next steps are going to be in developing better strategies to deal with
your innate temperament.

Being a highly sensitive man means being more sensitive to your
environment than other less sensitive men. Less sensitive men can,
of course, also be sensitive, and there are many situations in which
highly sensitive men can be very insensitive, particularly when they're
feeling overstimulated and stressed. In these kinds of situations, even
highly sensitive men can be unreasonable, temperamental, critical,
angry, annoyed, and impatient—just like any man. But at the same
time, their tendency and their pattern of generally being more sensitive to events, experiences, situations, people, and their environment
than less sensitive men will still be clearly evident.

This tendency can manifest itself in all areas of your life—your
relationships, your career, your free time, your preferences, your hobbies, your sense of yourself, and the relationship that you have with
yourself. It is likely that you do not experience your high sensitivity
as something that is constantly problematic in all areas of your life.
At the same time, it runs like a thread through your life, even if you
are only now for the first time able to put a name to it and to understand your emotional reactions and the pattern of behavior that is
related to your temperament. And it doesn't make any difference
whether you belong to the 30 percent of highly sensitive men who
are extroverted or the majority, the 70 percent of highly sensitive
men who are introverted in social settings.

All of these things will continue to be part of your life to some extent because you cannot completely get rid of your highly sensitive
temperament, nor can you "train it away." But you don't have to. What
you do have the power to do is to change your relationship with your
high sensitivity and the way you deal with it in your daily life. You do
not need to judge your temperament negatively or positively, but you
do have to accept it. The sooner that you are able to accept your tem-

peramental disposition, the better for you and for your quality of life because life is going to become much simpler and more pleasant. Simpler because, assuming that you have been rejecting this part of your personality, you will be able to free yourself from this struggle, from this rejection of a central part of your being, and in doing so, you will be able to deal with life in a freer and more flexible way.

In my work as a psychotherapist, I often notice that the cause of people's suffering and of many of their problems is the opposite of acceptance, that is to say, rejecting, not accepting, not wanting to have something. The psychiatrist and Gestalt therapist Arnold Beisser summarized the importance of acceptance in allowing change to begin in his paradoxical theory of change: "Change occurs when one becomes what he is, not when he tries to become what he is not."[1]

The reason that I think this quote is so applicable here is that it is exactly this approach that is going to be critical for you in dealing with your own high sensitivity. If you can accept that you get overstimulated more quickly or react more emotionally than most other men, instead of struggling against it, then you will have already made a fundamental change. It is only through the freedom that you can find in acceptance that you are going to be able to make positive changes. But if you desperately try to be different from how you actually are, then you will only create more suffering and more pressure in your life.

This is why I want to impress on you the importance of starting the process of self-acceptance. Now. When you begin to be able to accept yourself as you are, you are going to take the next step almost automatically, starting to adapt your lifestyle to your sensitive temperament and starting to enjoy it. Allow yourself the freedom to be who you are. You don't need to be different; you simply need to learn to accept who you have always been.

I'm going to be talking about the importance of acceptance a lot in this book because I have the feeling that very many, though not all, highly sensitive men grow up with the feeling that they are "not right," "not okay," or "not enough of a man" because of their high sensitivity. I believe that this can have wide-reaching, often lifelong consequences for your self-worth, your self-image, and your path in life. But whatever your experiences have been to date, you can achieve fundamental change in your life through self-acceptance.

Let's imagine your disposition as a garden. Where your garden is, the direction that the garden is facing, whether north, east, south, or west, is a given and cannot be changed. Of course, we can fertilize the soil and aerate it, but we can't plant a north-facing garden in the same way as we can plant a south-facing garden. But the moment we get to know our garden and understand what kind of garden it is, then we can begin to make plans and buy exactly the right flowers and plants that are going to thrive in this particular garden. Only then will we be able to enjoy our garden. And if we feel envious of our neighbor's garden because it seems to be in a better position than ours, then we're not going to enjoy our own garden for what it is. We're not going to see what makes our garden unique, what it offers us, what it needs to become a really beautiful garden.

Common Everyday Challenges for Highly Sensitive Men

What are the biggest challenges that highly sensitive men face in everyday life? Despite the fact that there are many different varieties of highly sensitive men in the world and I want to avoid generalizing here, there are number of problematic areas that I've noticed cropping up time and again over the years for my highly sensitive male clients.

1. OVERSTIMULATION AND INTENSE EMOTIONS

Highly sensitive men often find it unpleasant and sometimes even restricting that they become quickly overstimulated and stressed, often coupled with a lot of thoughts and intense feelings.

On the one hand, many men would like to feel "calmer, more laid back and relaxed," particularly in highly stimulating situations. On the other, many men would also like to be able to deal with their feelings differently in terms of how they identify them (what am I feeling?), interpret them (what's this feeling like?), express them (can I verbalize this feeling?), and regulate them (can I influence this feeling or even change it?). The skill here is to be able to address one's feelings, to learn to deal with these feelings, and to understand them, but at the same time not to allow oneself to be controlled by every feeling all of the time. In other words, highly sensitive men need to become very good at calming themselves down and regulating their intense emotions.

2. PROBLEMS WITH SELF-WORTH AND A LACK OF SELF-ACCEPTANCE

As mentioned above, a common feeling expressed among many highly sensitive men is the recurrent sense that they "are not okay," "aren't manly enough," or are in some way "inferior" to less sensitive men. This is often coupled with a range of negative judgments and underlying beliefs about one's self (e.g., "I am not worthy of love," "I'm not tough enough," "I'm too sensitive," "I'm too soft," etc.), a tendency to be very self-critical, and a recurring sense of shame. Many highly sensitive men have often experienced very *explicit* criticisms from other men in their lives, such as fathers who at worst rejected their sensitive "sissy" of a son and at best were simply unable to appreciate their sensitivity. Highly sensitive men may also have been bullied and shamed. I'm thinking here of fathers who call their sons "weaklings" or tell them that they need to "toughen up," or of classmates who tell their friends that they're acting "like a girl." What is also common is young highly sensitive men receiving countless *implicit* criticisms—an unspoken sense from the people around them that they're "different" from other boys. This is a subtle form of rejection and one that is often not directly verbalized. This can be something like being sidelined or picked last in team sports because you're more cautious and restrained than other boys. Or the angry silence of a parent because his highly sensitive son is crying. Although unspoken, these messages are received loud and clear and are often internalized.

The key is for highly sensitive men to know their worth and to value their strengths, of which there are many.

3. LACK OF SELF-CARE: LEADING A LIFESTYLE THAT DOESN'T SUIT YOUR TEMPERAMENT

Because people differ in their environmental sensitivity and because the majority of people in the world are not highly sensitive, many of the things that influence our daily lives are not necessarily "high-sensitivity friendly." Highly sensitive people are a minority; that's not an easy thing in itself, and it's connected with its own emotional strain. Social ideals and norms tend to be determined and prescribed by the majority. This means that highly sensitive men, whether consciously or unconsciously, often try to live up to the majority's demands in a way that tallies with the lives of men with a less sensitive disposition. The consequence of this is often a lifestyle that doesn't fit one's actual temperament, whether it be in the office, at home, in the family, or among social contacts. In many highly sensitive men, this can lead to discontentment, irritability, exhaustion, unhealthy behaviors (such as drug and alcohol misuse in an attempt to reduce the tension one feels), a feeling of chronic tension, or even anxious and depressive feelings.

The things that we can develop to deal with these issues include becoming better at looking after ourselves (self-care), becoming better at expressing our emotional needs and personal boundaries in respect to other people, allowing ourselves more time out and more quiet times, and making concrete changes in our lives that allow us to feel that our own lives as highly sensitive men are truthful and authentic.

Questions About Typical Problem Areas in Our Everyday Lives

Before addressing these practical challenges in the second half of this book, I'd like you to think about whether these three problem areas— *overstimulation and intense emotions, self-worth and self-acceptance,* and *lifestyle and self-care*—manifest themselves in your own life. And if they do, what are the areas that you struggle with the most?

Let me ask you a few questions that might help you to think about these issues. There are no right or wrong answers here.

- When and in which situations do you feel overstimulated?
- How does this overstimulation feel to you?
- What effects does this feeling of overstimulation have on your everyday life?
- How do you feel when you find yourself in a male-dominated environment?
- How self-confident are you when you meet potential partners?
- How have other men in your life reacted to your sensitivity to date?
- How do you react to setbacks or failures in your life?
- How often do you feel ashamed of how emotional or sensitive you are?
- When was the last time that you told someone what you needed from them emotionally?
- How do you generally feel at work?
- Are you able to say no when people ask you to do something that you don't want to do or offer you something that you know you don't want?
- What do you use the most energy for in everyday life?
- Which concrete changes could you make to bring more peace into your life?
- Do you have the feeling that you spend enough time alone?

Take some time and quietly think about these questions, then maybe make some notes in response to them. Sometimes it helps just to put these initial thoughts about wanting to change into words, which might previously have only existed as vague ideas or assumptions.

There are, of course, a range of other challenges that can arise in everyday life that fall outside of these three problem areas, such as sensitivity to subtleties, which includes a high sensory sensitivity to smaller variations in things such as noises, light, smells, and temperature. However, in the case of this particular issue, most highly sensitive people seem to find good solutions to the problems, either changing or avoiding the situation by, for instance, wearing earplugs, moving to a quieter area of town, changing lighting, or only buying clothes made from particular materials.

The three problematic areas that I've outlined above—overstimulation and intense emotions, self-worth and self-acceptance, and lifestyle and self-care—are generally harder nuts to crack, having been a challenge over many years, often since adolescence or even childhood. In this case, it is rarer for people to quickly find simple creative solutions because the changes that are needed require a much longer process of reflection, which requires patience and courage.

What High Sensitivity Isn't— How It Differs from Psychological Disorders

As we arrive at the end of this chapter, let's think again about what high sensitivity is *not* and how you can differentiate it from a psychological disorder. As mentioned above, it is quite possible to be highly sensitive and to also be dealing with a psychological disorder. But high sensitivity itself is not a psychological problem.

How our society defines what counts as psychologically "well" and psychologically "unwell" is not always very consistent, is sometimes very subjective, and often shifts in the light of change in public opinion. Homosexuality, for instance, was officially considered a psychological illness in the United States until 1973, whereas the American Psychiatric Association did not classify social anxiety disorder (a fear of social situations) as an official diagnosis until 1980. Nevertheless, we can broadly say that when we're talking about a psychological disorder, we're generally referring to a collection of cognitive (perception, memory, thought), emotional, and behavioral symptoms that put a person under serious psychological strain and that are accompanied by impairments in social, professional, or other important functional areas.

It is not always easy having a particularly sensitive nature, and there may well be specific everyday situations in which it feels like a real challenge or disadvantage, but this doesn't necessarily lead to serious psychological strain or impairments in how you function. It is important to understand this.

Psychologically healthy highly sensitive people are just as resilient in the face of challenges as less sensitive people. The decisive difference here is how the challenges manifest themselves. Let's look at a concrete example. It is completely possible that a highly sensitive man who finds himself working in an environment that is a bad fit for him may start to experience feelings of depression, exhaustion, and mood swings, whereas a man who is not highly sensitive may find the same working environment unproblematic and may remain completely psychologically healthy. At the same time, it's not the man's highly sensitive temperament that is automatically making him sick, because in a working environment that was a good fit for his temperament he would be thriving. Remember, the fact that a man is more sensitive to his environment means that he also reacts better to positive stimuli, experiences, and events. And this is an important part of our psychological resilience. I also believe that having a higher level of sensitivity and reactivity to your environment can, in fact, protect you against psychological illness because highly sensitive people register more quickly than others when something in their environment isn't right or isn't doing them any good. This is an important prerequisite for being able to modify our behavior—whether it be at work, in our relationships, or when making decisions.

Sometimes clients come to my practice because they've read about high sensitivity, they recognize it in themselves, and they believe that it explains the difficulties that they've been experiencing. But when we explore their problems over the course of a few sessions, we often discover that while they may also be highly sensitive, they are, in fact, suffering from an acute psychological disorder that requires urgent treatment. It is often the case that I can't detect all of the DOES indicators in the client and that I don't recognize any of the classic signs of high sensitivity in the client's behavior. Instead, what is clear is that this person is suffering from a serious psychological disorder but has convinced himself that he is "just highly sensitive." It would take too long to chronicle the differences between high sensitivity and each of the psychological disorders listed in the current edition of the World Health Organization's International Classification of Diseases (the eleventh revision, known as ICD-11).[2] Nevertheless, I would like to give you a brief overview of the psychological disorders that I believe are most often confused with high sensitivity.

Affective Disorders

The term *affective disorders* refers to psychological illnesses that manifest themselves in changes to one's mood, either as a depression—with or without anxiety—or as an elevated mood (mania or the more moderate hypomania).

A depressive episode is marked by a low mood, lack of energy, and the loss of concentration and interest in doing things. It is often accompanied by problems sleeping (such as waking up early), a loss of libido, a loss of self-confidence and appetite, and, at its most serious, thoughts about death and suicide.

As we know from the studies outlined earlier, highly sensitive people are only more prone to depression if they experienced a difficult childhood. When we compare the above description of the symptoms of depression with the characteristics and indicators of high sensitivity, the differences quickly become clear. It is true that both high sensitivity and depression can lead to people feeling thin-skinned, to a lack of self-confidence, and to a tendency to withdraw socially, but even here we need to differentiate between someone slowly developing a new tendency and someone having a general characteristic that has always been present. In other words, we need to separate between "state" and "trait." Thoughts of suicide, a lack of joy, and a feeling that one is unable to deal with daily activities are not signs of a temperamental trait, but are a clear indication of a serious psychological state or illness, such as a depressive episode.

Social Phobia

Social phobia, or social anxiety disorder, is an explicit fear of being the center of attention. This often leads to socially phobic people avoiding situations in which they fear that they may behave in an embarrassing or demeaning way. Social phobia is often connected with low self-esteem and a fear of criticism and being judged negatively by other people. It can lead to symptoms of anxiety, such as trembling, blushing, nausea, or a need to urinate more often than normal. It is marked by clear emotional stress brought on by both the symptoms of the anxiety and the avoidant behavior, and the symptoms are exclusively limited to the feared social situations and thoughts about these situations. We might think of social phobia as the big sister of shyness, which is, of course, not a pathological condition, or the more common stage fright, which most of us have experienced at some point in our lives.

As we already know, around two thirds of all highly sensitive people are introverted, and many of these people will also be shy if they suffered from negative experiences in their childhoods.[3] Combined with the fact that highly sensitive people react more quickly and more strongly to subtle stimuli, including social cues from other people, it is clear why highly sensitive behavior can be mistaken for socially anxious or shy behavior. It is also true that many highly sensitive people react with social anxiety in certain situations. And yet to make a diagnosis of social phobia as a psychological disorder, it must manifest itself as explicit emotional distress caused by the clearly defined symptoms of anxiety outlined above and the related avoidant behavior. Some people have posited the theory that high sensitivity, or sensory processing sensitivity, could represent a risk factor in the development of social phobia.[4] But more research is needed here to clearly define the relationship between high sensitivity and social phobia.

Post-Traumatic Stress Disorder

The IDC-10's definition of post-traumatic stress disorder (PTSD) is a "delayed or protracted response to a stressful event or situation (of either brief or long duration) of an exceptionally threatening or catastrophic nature, which is likely to cause pervasive distress in almost anyone."[5] Symptoms include intrusive memories in the form of flashbacks, dreams, or nightmares, feeling numb or emotionally desensitized, apathy, avoidance of activities and situations that might trigger memories of the trauma, but also a state of hypervigilance, excessive jumpiness, and problems sleeping. Anxiety and depression, as well as suicidal thoughts, are also common in people with PTSD.

Research into high sensitivity refers to the genetic component of sensitivity as an innate temperamental trait that has an evolutionary explanation and can already be observed in infancy. Even children who've experienced a "good" childhood without any notable problems or attachment issues still exhibit the characteristics of high sensitivity. This is a clear argument against the idea that high sensitivity—as defined by Aron—is the result of trauma. The symptoms of psychological sensitivity and arousal that go hand in hand with trauma were not apparent in people suffering with PTSD before they experienced the traumatic situation, and these psychological issues often manifest themselves in situations that mirror or are similar to the traumatic situation. This is not the case with high sensitivity, where the tendency to become overstimulated is spread much wider and has existed for much longer. And unlike highly sensitive people, traumatized people do not necessarily display increased empathy or a long-term tendency to process information more deeply.

Personality Disorders: Emotionally Unstable (Borderline Type), Anxious Avoidant, and Narcissistic Personality Disorders

Personality disorders are "severe disturbances in the personality and behavioral tendencies of the individual, . . . usually involving several areas of the personality; [are] nearly always associated with considerable personal distress and social disruption; [and] have usually manifested since childhood or adolescence and continue throughout adulthood."[6] There are a range of different types of personality disorders, but I want to start by focusing on the differences between high sensitivity and borderline personality disorder, which is marked by emotional instability, impulsiveness, problems with one's sense of self, a chronic sense of emptiness, and often self-destructive behavior. Despite the fact that highly sensitive men also have a tendency toward emotional intensity, we do not see the other clinical signs of borderline personality disorders in psychologically healthy highly sensitive people, such as high levels of anger, fear of abandonment, and impulsiveness. Highly sensitive people are usually the very opposite of impulsive.

If social phobia is the big sister of nonpathological shyness, then anxious avoidant personality disorder is the mother of both. Marked by chronic and wide-ranging tension and worry, the conviction that you are socially awkward, unattractive, or worthless, and the fear of being criticized or rejected in social situations, this disorder limits sufferers' lives, causing them to avoid professional and social activities because they are terrified of disapproval. There are similarities with high sensitivity, in that many highly sensitive men, for instance, have described to me feelings of low self-worth, the tendency to feel awkward and overstimulated in many social situations, and the tendency to withdraw. The difference here, though, is again the strength of the symptoms and the consistency with which the symptoms present themselves. It is also the case that highly sensitive people react with strong positive *and* negative emotions in all areas of life, and not only with anxious feelings in social situations in which one is at risk of being criticized. To add to this, sensitivity to subtle stimuli is not a diagnostic criterion in the case of anxious avoidant personality disorder.

I would like to finish by looking at narcissistic personality disorder. The symptoms that people with this disorder exhibit include an overblown but also fragile feeling of self-worth, a strong need to be admired and to be the center of attention, a sense of one's own greatness, and a lack of empathy for others. The parallel to people with high sensitivity here is in their sensitivity to criticism and rejection, which highly sensitive people also react strongly to. But beyond this, the presentation of these phenomena is very different, because high sensitivity goes hand in hand with a high degree of empathy, not a lack of it. Also, many highly sensitive people behave in an introverted, cautious, or sometimes even shy way, which is very different from the status-oriented, admiration- and attention-seeking behavior of narcissistic people. The avoidance of intimacy and vulnerability in relation to other people is typical for narcissists, while highly sensitive people often consciously seek out these things in their relationships and, indeed, need them to feel well, as they provide depth. A lack of depth in relationships tends to make highly sensitive people feel easily bored.

SUMMARY

As this chapter ends, I hope that you feel that you now have a good understanding of the typical problem areas for highly sensitive men—overstimulation and intense emotions, self-worth and self-acceptance, and lifestyle and self-care—and that you understand how these often crop up in daily life. It is also important to me that you now find it easier to differentiate high sensitivity from psychological disorders, although, of course, it is possible for a person to be highly sensitive *and* to be suffering from a mental health disorder. If that is the case for you, then it is vital that you adequately deal with the acute psychological illness first. When your psychological health has stabilized or improved, then you can begin to address your sensitive temperament.

Before we move on to the second half of this book, in which we'll talk about the best ways of dealing practically with these typical problem areas, I'd like to invite you to take another look at any notes that you made during this chapter and to think about what the biggest challenge is for you about being highly sensitive.

Toby: "We are all still stuck with the strong, macho, insensitive caveman image of masculinity, despite some superficial efforts to convince us otherwise."

Toby is in his mid forties, is married, and has three kids. Here he talks openly about how his high sensitivity has helped him interact with women and deepened his sexuality. His observations about cultural differences are very interesting, as is the fact that he has witnessed how particularly sensitive men are having a hard time in most cultures.

When and how did you first notice you were highly sensitive?

I have always known that I was "different" from others, but I really discovered the term *highly sensitive* when I was recovering from my second burnout a few years ago. My therapist at that time recommended some books to me, and that led me to read about Elaine Aron's work. I did an HSP questionnaire online and that got the ball rolling.

What are the advantages and the disadvantages of being highly sensitive?

I have never felt that sensitive men are generally accepted in our society, so the advantages are very limited, in my view. When I grew up, every man who wasn't tough was called a pussy, sissy, or fag. Being sensitive was unacceptable. We are all still stuck with the strong, macho, insensitive caveman image of masculinity, despite some superficial efforts to convince us otherwise. Any sensitivity in a man is still seen as a "weakness," and that is the main disadvantage of being highly sensitive, in my opinion. When you mention to others that you're highly sensitive, you get automatically labeled as "weak and soft." A follower, not a leader. A pushover, not a fighter. I think that can be a problem in particular in the professional world, and some might fail to see the huge asset a highly sensitive person could be to their team, as such people often think deeply, are innovative, and are particularly good at problem-solving and being creative. So all these qualities go to waste.

I think other advantages are being able to connect with others on an emotional and intellectual level and working well in a one-to-one setting, particularly with women and children.

How does your high sensitivity impact on your relationships with other men?

I have very few close relationships with other men, except with my son and my father-in-law. All other male relationships I have usually remain superficial. I often feel that other men don't want to share personal or emotional issues and remain reserved or find my being open threatening. As long as it's all "Yo—look at that chick, pass me the beer," it's all good, but when you mention feelings, a lot of men close up like a clam. I have the sense that they often have no idea how to handle me or how to respond.

How does your high sensitivity impact on your relationships with women?

My relationships with women are often very good, whether they are of an intimate and sexual nature or not. I can tap into their way of feeling and thinking, and they really seem to appreciate my ability of being able to do so. I have experienced very little hostility or rejection from women, but have been asked on a few occasions whether I was gay. When it comes to sexuality, I think I'm very good at tuning in to what the woman wants and can react accordingly, with satisfying results for both of us.

What are the challenges of being a highly sensitive father?

I want to use my abilities to connect with my children, who range from "normally" sensitive, to more sensitive, to highly sensitive, and I regularly succeed at doing so. However, often my own difficult upbringing interferes with this. Everything about children is completely new to me, and I have no references I could fall back on. It really is learning on the job without guidelines, yet so far I seem to be doing pretty well, given the good relationship I have with my children.

One very important issue I have tackled with them is bringing up sensitive issues like sex, first relationships, mental and physical changes during puberty, and so forth. By being able to almost immediately sense their apprehension in bringing up subjects like this, I can make it easier for them by taking the first step or by gently steering the conversation in the right direction. By doing so, we can discuss anything openly, and hopefully, I can answer their questions.

What are the advantages and the disadvantages of being highly sensitive at work?

Noting very small behavioral changes or pointing out something that was amiss, both with victims and suspects, was something I often used to my advantage when I was working as a law enforcement officer. Right now I work with adolescent boys who are refugees. Due to my sensitivity, I sense when something is wrong with them. I can get them to open up fairly easily and often sense underlying emotions when they talk—the anger, the fear, the pain, the constant loneliness. I shudder just thinking about some of their stories. I often use myself as an example, show them I dare to open up, and they often follow suit, despite their backgrounds often interfering. The ability to really listen to people, being able to detect where the real issue is and being able to reflect on that and respond appropriately, is definitely a strength at work that is linked to my sensitivity.

You work with people with diverse cultural backgrounds; is high sensitivity dealt with differently in different communities?

I have had the opportunity to work and live all over the world, interacting with people from many different cultures, and overall, I haven't seen much of a difference in how men with high sensitivity are treated and regarded. I do believe the world would be a much better place if we used the qualities associated with high sensitivity better.

What's your advice for other highly sensitive men?

Find yourself, know yourself, stay true to yourself. Stand your ground and demand rest and solitude when needed.

PART II

Living (Well) as a Highly Sensitive Man

Strategies to Deal With Overstimulation and Intense Emotions: What Emotional Regulation Is and Why It Matters for Highly Sensitive Men

HAVING A VERY SENSITIVE NERVOUS system means that highly sensitive men often become quickly overstimulated. They process internal stimuli more deeply (feelings, thoughts, bodily sensations) as well as external stimuli (people, noises, light, smells), which can quickly lead to them feeling overaroused. This state of overstimulation can then manifest itself in the form of strong feelings, disparate thoughts, physical, mental, and emotional tension, and an inner restlessness. This is often followed by exhaustion and tiredness, because your nervous system has been running "on overdrive." As outlined in the last chapter, this is often the biggest challenge about being highly sensitive, alongside issues around self-worth and a lack of self-awareness, as well as how we manage our lifestyles. So I now want to introduce you to a number of strategies to regulate your emotions that are going to help you to become much better at dealing with overstimulation and intense emotions.

And then, in the remaining chapters of the book, I'm going to address self-worth, self-acceptance, and how we can learn to lead a self-caring and "high-sensitivity-friendly" life.

The tendency to become overstimulated can't be completely avoided because it's impossible to steer clear of all potentially challenging situations—be it a visit to a busy supermarket, your brother's birthday party, giving a presentation at work, organizing or booking your next vacation, or an upcoming parents' evening about how well your kids are doing at school. All of these situations can quickly feel overstimulating because they are accompanied by the processing of numerous internal and external stimuli. It is thus not possible to completely avoid overstimulation, not least because it would likely cause you to lead a very controlled and boring life. In order to lead an active life, take risks, pursue life goals, and experience new things, it is sometimes worth accepting short bouts of overstimulation. And at the end of the day, although overstimulation feels unpleasant, it is only a problem for your health if you remain in a chronic state of overstimulation without ever giving your nervous system a break.

The challenge for someone who has a tendency to become overstimulated and to feel things very strongly—which are often experienced together—is learning to deal with these feelings whenever possible. This means that highly sensitive men need to get much better at calming themselves down when they notice that they feel overstimulated, tense, or very emotional. Emotional regulation can really help with this. In the context of psychotherapy, emotional regulation is the ability to change and regulate your own feelings, particularly when these feelings are very intense and unpleasant. The goal here isn't to not feel anything anymore or just to feel good, but rather to get better at tolerating our feelings and emotional arousal so that we don't feel helplessly controlled by them. The following emotional regulation skills can help us deal better with overstimulation and intense feelings:

- The ability to notice, differentiate, and name your emotions ("I feel angry," "I feel upset," "I feel cross").
- The ability to recognize triggers and maintaining factors for your emotions ("I feel ... because ...," "Whenever I do ..., then I feel ...").
- The ability to influence the intensity, duration, and quality of emotions.
- The development of mindfulness and acceptance when dealing with emotions. (observing feelings before taking action, learning to tolerate feelings; instead of saying "I want/must/should not feel this way," learning to say "I feel ...,at the moment, and that's OK" or "I feel ..., and I'm going to keep observing this feeling until it changes").
- Learning to normalize emotions ("It's normal and not a problem to feel like this," "Other people feel like this in these sort of situations").
- Learning to better recognize the connection between basic emotional needs and emotions ("I feel better in this moment because ...," "When I feel ..., then I need ...").
- When you do experience negative emotions, learning to be supportive and caring in relation to yourself, empathizing with yourself and confronting your own suffering or pain in a kind and compassionate way, just as you would with a friend ("I'm there for you," "This isn't easy for you," "I can feel your pain," "You're not alone, I'm here with you," "Tell me what's wrong").
- Learning to form alternative, self-calming thoughts ("Stay calm," "Take this slowly," "One step at a time").
- The ability to make concrete changes to your behavior in different situations (i.e., consciously doing something differently or specifically doing something to calm yourself or to make the situation better or more tolerable for yourself).

- The use of physical relaxation techniques (relaxing your body, muscles, and breathing when you're feeling tense or stressed).
- Getting better at using your imagination (for instance, recalling past events and situations that gave you strength and made you feel calm, relaxed, and secure, or recalling a calming location or a trusted person whom you associate with positive feelings and memories).

The skills we use to regulate our feelings—which we usually use completely automatically and unconsciously in our daily lives—are things that we learn very early on in life, as infants and children, through our contact with our parents. Our parents also present us with a direct model of how we might deal with our feelings, which we learn and internalize. The good news is that whatever we experienced as children, whatever our model was, by consciously using the strategies outlined above, we can still strengthen and develop our ability to regulate and change our feelings in later life. At the same time, we also now know that deficits in emotional regulation, in terms of the way we perceive, designate, tolerate, understand, and modify our feelings, can cause and sustain psychological problems.

The German psychiatrist Claas-Hinrich Lammers wrote, "The ability to successfully adapt and regulate one's emotions has a demonstrably positive influence on our health, our relationships, and our professional success. Difficulties with the adaptive regulation and processing of emotions, on the other hand, are both a causative and maintaining factor in psychological illnesses."[1]

This is why emotional regulation is so important and why recent psychotherapeutic developments in cognitive behavioral therapy, known as the third-wave of cognitive behavioral therapy, all have a strongly emotionally focused approach.

But why is emotional regulation particularly important for people who are highly sensitive? An Australian study looking into the link between high sensitivity and emotional regulation found that highly sensitive people are more conscious of their negative feelings than less sensitive people, but that they also find it harder to regulate their emotions.[2] The study highlighted that it was people's failure to accept difficult feelings that played a decisive role here, as well as a sense that they couldn't change or influence these unpleasant feelings. This all means that you, as a highly sensitive man, need to become a real expert in dealing with your feelings and calming yourself down. You also need to strengthen your belief in your own ability to regulate your emotions, which you're going to learn in the rest of this book.

Let's think back to the "orchid children" we heard about in chapter 2 and the babies who were "slow to warm up" and "behaviorally inhibited." All of these different terms from different studies all basically describe the same thing: a heightened sensitivity and reactivity to one's environment. When exposed to new experiences, these kids exhibit stronger symptoms of stress than other kids in the form of raised muscular tension and a raised heart rate, while their behavior remains cautious, observant, reserved, or inhibited. If you identify today as a highly sensitive man, then you were also a highly sensitive baby and little boy. And if you cried as a baby because, perhaps, you were overtired, then it was probably your parents or another guardian who (hopefully) tried to comfort you and calm you down. Of course, this isn't always the case, but ideally, they did this by holding you in their arms, stroking you, speaking to you in a gentle voice, or singing or humming; they touched you or distracted you in order to help you calm down and reduce your emotional and physical tension.

And this is, in effect, exactly what you can do as a highly sensitive adult man when you find yourself in a state of emotional overstimulation. You wouldn't have calmed down or stopped crying when you were a baby or a child if your parents had shouted at you, criticized you, or left you in a room on your own. So it's vital that in difficult moments you are able to use emotional regulation to look after yourself and comfort yourself instead of criticizing your tendency to become quickly overstimulated and to feel things intensely ("Oh, here we go again!") This only increases the tension you feel and your emotional arousal and doesn't help you calm down more quickly.

What Are Emotions?

If we're going to talk about regulating emotions and why this is so important for highly sensitive people, then I think it's important to define exactly what we mean when we use the term *emotions*. In everyday usage, the terms *emotion* and *feeling* are used synonymously to describe our emotional state. I have also done that in this book, although a feeling is, in fact, just a part of an emotion. "I feel sad," "I'm excited," "I'm afraid," "I'm so furious I could explode"—all of these phrases describe emotional states. The psychologist Paul Ekman empirically established seven *basic emotions*, which can be recognized in different cultures, are biologically set, and are already present during the first years of our lives. These are enjoyment, anger, disgust, fear, contempt, sadness, and surprise.[3] All of our other emotions develop from these basic emotions into what are known as our *social emotions*, which include guilt, shame, and jealousy.

Lammers describes the term *emotion* as follows: "An emotion is an acute and temporary intuitive, physiological, behavioral, and cognitive reaction to an individually meaningful event."[4]

In other words, an emotion is experienced on many different levels, all of which are connected with each other and automatically and permanently influence each other. Let's take the emotion of fear as an example. A job interview is a situation that many of us will have experienced and felt nervous about, and the emotion of fear might have manifested itself as follows:

- **FEELING:** Fear, nervousness, panic
- **BODY:** Shallow breathing, muscle tension, sweating, increased blood pressure, increased heart rate, rigid facial expression, dry mouth

- **THOUGHTS:** "Just don't get anything wrong," "I really hope I get this job," "The boss is looking really serious"
- **BEHAVIOR:** Being attentive, answering questions in a comprehensive way, shifting about on your chair, trying to laugh despite feeling tense inside

The fact that these four different areas influence each other is advantageous for us because it means that we can work on all four areas in order to calm ourselves down or to make the situation more tolerable. We can try to accept and recognize our *feeling* of fear (which doesn't mean that we have to like it) by saying, for instance, "I feel scared in this moment. That's OK. Fear comes and goes." We can try to calm our *body* by breathing deeply and relaxing our muscles. We can try to formulate alternative, helpful, and self-calming *thoughts*, such as, "Stay calm. This isn't an easy situation. You're doing fine. You can tolerate this fear. Your last job interview went well even though you were nervous." And we can modify our *behavior* to influence how we feel in a given situation. We can have a sip of water, for instance, change our sitting position, or ask a question. All of these things can help us reduce the intensity of our feeling of fear and help us tolerate the way that we feel in that situation.

These four categories can also help illuminate overstimulation caused by too much internal or external stimulation. My impression is that overstimulation is often connected with strong feelings, although this isn't always the case. Sometimes clients tell me that they have felt very overstimulated without being able to link it to a specific feeling. Most highly sensitive men that I have met know the feeling of overstimulation very well and know exactly which situations usually trigger it. But others find it harder to recognize overstimulation and tend instead to describe it as an "unpleasant state," as "stress" or as "an internal tension and restlessness." One client told me that for him, overstimulation meant "at first having too many thoughts," followed by having "an empty head," which he connected with a feeling "that everything is too much." The following exercises are going to help you get better at recognizing the signs of overstimulation in yourself.

Recognizing the Signs of Overstimulation

What are the signs of overstimulation for you personally?

- Typical situations or triggering events (who, what, when, where?):

  _____

  _____

- Feeling (rated in intensity from 0 to 100):

  _____

  _____

- Thoughts that trigger or accompany my feelings:

  _____

  _____

- Physical sensations and physical changes:

  _____

  _____

- Behavior or behavioral impulses (what would you like to do in the situation?)

  _____

  _____

The sooner that you can recognize when you are in a state of overstimulation, the quicker you will be able to respond to it. All four categories—thoughts, feelings, body, and behavior—offer different opportunities for calming yourself down and regulating your emotions. The first step is often just naming and acknowledging your own feelings ("In this moment, I feel . . . ") because this is an emotional regulation skill in itself, which can help us feel that we have more control and have created the necessary distance to deal with the feeling. When we have a concrete name for a feeling, then it becomes much easier to address it and it feels less diffused and less threatening. To add to this, being able to name our feelings helps us to discover which emotional needs are being expressed by that feeling.

Recognizing Emotions and the Needs That Underlie Them

I often tell my highly sensitive clients that we don't need to be afraid of our emotions, even the unpleasant ones, because they represent a great source of information. Of course, this is easier said than done because in the first instance we all try to avoid negative or unpleasant feelings. Who enjoys feeling sad, helpless, or lonely? But sometimes there are irrational beliefs behind our fear of unpleasant feelings, such as, "If I let this feeling in, it's never going to stop." This is a belief that we need to consciously recognize and challenge.

A feeling is like a wave that comes and goes. It is never permanent, despite the fact that we're often afraid that it will be. And at the same time, the broad spectrum of our feelings, including the unpleasant ones, is what makes our lives and human existence so lively, interesting, and diverse. We would often rather not experience the negative or unpleasant feelings in life and just experience the positive or pleasant ones, but at the end of the day they're two sides of the same coin. The one cannot exist without the other. All of our feelings are important and have a function. Even the grief that we feel after the death of a loved one is necessary because it shows us that that person was important to us and that our relationship with that person had meaning in our life, that life itself is meaningful to us. Feelings enrich our life, spur us into action, and encourage us to do things. They give our lives meaning. What would life even be without feelings? The complexity of our emotions and the thoughts connected to them are what make us human. And yet we are often afraid of what we feel.

One way of learning to fear our own feelings less, of developing a less "emotion-phobic" attitude to life, is to recognize that our feelings are giving us important information about what our emotional needs are in a given situation and about whether these needs are being satisfied, frustrated, or apparently threatened. We know from psychology that human beings have numerous basic emotional needs, which all need to be adequately satisfied. As such, they are of central importance if we want to develop and maintain our psychological health. The German psychologist Klaus Grawe posited four basic emotional needs, which, he believed, all of us try to satisfy and which are bound up with our psychological health.[5] They are:

- **NEED FOR ATTACHMENT:** Feeling secure, safe, and emotionally close to others, for instance, to our parents, friends, partners, or children.
- **NEED FOR ORIENTATION AND CONTROL:** Not feeling helpless, but feeling that we are able to determine, form, and change our own lives and living conditions, for example, by making decisions, acting self-autonomously, taking control, saying no.
- **NEED TO INCREASE AND PROTECT OUR SELF-WORTH:** Feeling that one has worth as a human being, for instance, feeling valuable or self-confident, feeling proud, being praised, experiencing professional or personal success.
- **NEED FOR PLEASURE:** Taking part in activities that are connected to fun, pleasure, joy, or fulfillment while avoiding activities that are unpleasant or disagreeable, for instance, pursuing hobbies and interests, taking part in pleasant activities, playing, feeling sexually fulfilled, experiencing joy, experiencing meaning.

The emergence of feelings and emotions, whether positive or negative, can be traced back to the satisfaction of, frustration of, or potential threat to these four basic needs, in their myriad different manifestations in different people. Satisfying any of these emotional needs too little is just as problematic as satisfying them too much.

Let's take a concrete example. How did you feel yesterday evening? Relieved? Loved? Lonely? Envious? Annoyed? It was probably a mix of different feelings, but there was also probably a feeling that dominated. If you can start by naming that concrete feeling, then you'll be able to think about which of your basic emotional needs were being expressed through this feeling and whether this need was being satisfied, frustrated, or potentially threatened. Were you surrounded by loved ones and did you feel safe and understood in their presence (satisfaction of your need for attachment)? Did you have a productive day at work and feel that you'd done a good job (satisfaction of your need for self-worth)? Were you at the movies eating popcorn and laughing at a film (satisfaction of your need for pleasure)? Did you make a decision and feel free and clear-headed after making it (satisfaction of your need for control)? Or were you home alone, feeling lonely and sad (frustration of your need for attachment)?

The ability to recognize the connection between our feelings and our emotional needs can really help us to get rid of our discomfort or even fear of our own feelings, because we will begin to realize that these feelings aren't coming out of nowhere. Our emotional life can seem less senseless, threatening, or random and can motivate us to make changes to our behavior aimed at fulfilling our emotional needs. Instead of just feeling unwell, we can think, "I feel lonely (feeling) because I was home alone the whole day (frustrated emotional need for attachment). So I'm going to call a friend and organize a meet-up (need-oriented behavioral change)."

You can see from the examples above that it's really important that we are able to define our feelings. It can help us to understand what our emotional needs are and show us what we need in life or in a particular situation or phase of life, so that we can feel good or understand which of the four basic emotional needs we are getting too little or too much of. In other words, our feelings help us to

understand ourselves better. They are important signposts for potential changes that we can make to our behavior. Of course, our
feelings are not always going to be right, and I don't believe that we
should always listen to our feelings, but they can give us a huge
amount of information that we should be paying attention to.

The next exercises are going to help you get better at naming your
own feelings. As already mentioned, this is in itself a really important
strategy for regulating emotions. Lammers put together the following list of emotions to help us define more clearly what we're feeling.[6]

Recognizing Our Emotions

Try to sense which of the following feelings you're feeling today
most strongly. Sometimes we will sense a mixture of feelings. Over
the next few days, look at the following list regularly to help you
work out which feelings you are feeling most strongly on each day.

Abandonment	Contentment	Embarrassment
Admiration	Contrariness	Empathy
Adoration	Curiosity	Emptiness
Affection	Dejection	Enthusiasm
Amazement	Delight	Envy
Amusement	Desire	Euphoria
Anger	Disappointment	Excitement
Annoyance	Disbelief	Exhilaration
Aversion	Discontent	Exuberance
Awe	Discord	Fear
Benevolence	Discouragement	Frustration
Boredom	Disgust	Fury
Cheer	Dismay	Gratitude
Cluelessness	Displeasure	Grief
Coldness	Disquiet	Guilt
Contempt	Doubt	Happiness

Hatred	Offense	Shame
Homesickness	Pain	Shock
Hope	Panic	Sorrow
Hopelessness	Passion	Surprise
Humiliation	Pleasure	Sympathy
Impatience	Pressure	Tempestuousness
Insecurity	Pride	Tenderness
Irritability	Pugnacity	Tension
Irritation	Rage	Triumph
Jealousy	Rancor	Trust
Joy	Regret	Warmth
Loathing	Relief	Weariness
Loneliness	Reluctance	Wellness
Longing	Remorse	Wistfulness
Love	Resentment	Wonder
Lust	Restlessness	Worry
Melancholy	Sadness	Yearning
Mistrust	Schadenfreude	

Most people can say whether they feel good, bad, or okay, but they often find it difficult to differentiate their feelings any further, despite the fact that when we see a list of emotions like this we suddenly realize how many there actually are. It might be really helpful to practice this exercise of observing and naming your feelings over a longer period, such as a couple of days. The next exercise builds on the last one and expands it to help us think about the kinds of thoughts that arise in specific situations.

Emotion Journal

I would like to suggest that you start keeping an emotion journal to help you strengthen your ability to recognize your own emotions. Over the next week, write down what your strongest feeling is on

	SITUATION (WHO, WHAT, WHEN, WHERE?)	THOUGHT (WHAT WAS GOING THROUGH MY HEAD?)	FEELING (0–100) (WHAT DID I FEEL AND HOW STRONG WAS THAT FEELING?)
MONDAY			
TUESDAY			
WEDNESDAY			
THURSDAY			
FRIDAY			
SATURDAY			
SUNDAY			

each day (anger, exuberance, mistrust, etc.) and how intensively you experienced that feeling (ranking it in intensity from 0 to 100, with 100 indicating the highest level of intensity). Also write down, as precisely as possible, the concrete thoughts that triggered or accompanied that feeling (for instance, "This is never going to work!") and in which situation the feeling came up (who, what, when, where?). You can record both positive and negative feelings. If you find it difficult to name your feelings, you can use the list of emotions from the last task to help you define them.

If you can keep up this emotion journal for several weeks, then you'll begin to notice that your ability to observe and name your feelings is going to get stronger and stronger. The following exercise expands this concept to encompass your emotional needs and will improve your ability to use your emotions as a source of information about your needs.

Analysis of Needs

Over the next few weeks, begin to try to notice the connection between your feelings and your underlying emotional needs. Which emotional need is being frustrated, satisfied, or threatened and thus expressed through your feeling? On each day, note the feeling that you experienced most strongly on that day. This can be either a pleasant or an unpleasant feeling. Think about which emotional need might be reflected in this feeling (for instance, attachment, control, self-worth, or pleasure) and whether this need is being frustrated or satisfied, or whether you perceive that it is under threat in the

	SITUATION	FEELING (0–100)	EMOTIONAL NEED
MONDAY			
TUESDAY			
WEDNESDAY			
THURSDAY			
FRIDAY			
SATURDAY			
SUNDAY			

situation. Your emotional need in the particular situation may, of course, sit in the grey areas between the four basic emotional needs outlined above, manifesting perhaps as a need for support, security, clarity, recognition, confirmation, success, ease, encouragement, affection, or pleasure.

Once you are able to recognize how you feel and what your emotional needs in a given situation are, then you'll also find it easier to judge whether the feeling and the emotional need connected to it are appropriate and, if not, to be able to consider what a healthier way of dealing with both might look like. When we know what we need emotionally in a given moment, we can go on to think about what we could change (behavior, body, thoughts, or feelings) to bring us closer to fulfilling this emotional need. Do I need to change my behavior? Do I need to confront myself in a loving way and support myself mentally? Do I need to be brave? Do I need to relax my body or breathe particularly deeply? Do I need to accept the situation and this feeling and wait until something changes? Or do I need to recall an earlier situation when I was able to tolerate this same feeling? When we're too hot, we react to this physical feeling and our need to cool off by taking off our sweater or opening the window. When we're hungry or thirsty, we eat or drink. Why don't we do the same thing when we're dealing with our emotions?

SUMMARY

Of course, no one is constantly emotionally well-regulated all of the time and knows in every moment of their lives what they're thinking and feeling. I also think it's impossible to have all of your emotional needs fulfilled all of the time. Despite this, though, it is really worth addressing our feelings and the needs that sit behind them because it will help us to better understand ourselves.

In this chapter, I aimed to explain to you what emotional regulation means and why the ability to regulate our emotions is so important for you as a highly sensitive man. If you become better at dealing with your feelings and you're able to reduce your high level of arousal more quickly, then this is going to represent a very essential protective tool for you. The first step to better emotional regulation is being able to name your own feelings and to recognize the connection between your emotions and your core emotional needs. Now that you've completed these first exercises, you've already begun to strengthen your ability to regulate your emotions. In the next chapter, we're going to look at some more strategies in which we're going to use mindfulness and acceptance to regulate our feelings and calm ourselves down.

Henry: "It was only when I began to see my own self-worth that I began to feel as if I was accepted by other men as a highly sensitive man."

Henry is in his late thirties, currently single, and works in strategic communication. He is a gay man who is also highly sensitive, and so offers us an important perspective on masculine identity and diversity. Contrary to old stereotypes about gay men, he finds no-strings-attached, promiscuous sex difficult, something that many of my heterosexual highly sensitive clients have also told me when talking about their sex lives. This strongly suggests to me that it is largely temperament, rather than sexual orientation, that actually makes a difference in how we express ourselves sexually.

When and how did you first notice you were highly sensitive?

As far as my conscious memories go, even in my very early childhood I was always somehow a "special" kid who enjoyed being in the presence of others, but also needed to be on my own just as much. Back then I thought it was because I just enjoyed thinking or reading, but now I know it was basically a need to process all the external input that I got. I remember throughout the whole of my childhood and youth, my parents had to "pull" me out of the house so that I would spend time with my peers because I preferred to be in my own world—with my books, writing, studying astronomy. I also enjoyed the company of animals because they seemed to understand me, and I understood them, without any hassle or unnecessary talking.

In my teenage years, when, of course, I wanted to be with my peers, I learned to numb my senses with alcohol, which made it bearable for me to be out, have fun with others, and feel like I belonged somewhere. I always had a very bizarre feeling of being so different from everyone else, and I always wanted to be like them so much. It was also very difficult for me to get to know new people, so I preferred to be close to a few selected friends and withdraw (if not physically, then at least mentally) from the crowd.

But all that was when I didn't know that I was highly sensitive. I thought I was just "wrong." I only learned about the concept of high sensitivity recently, and it has brought about a substantial change in my understanding of the world around me and, most importantly, myself.

What are the advantages and the disadvantages of being highly sensitive?

I think there are several advantages of being highly sensitive: a higher sensitivity and empathy, which help me to understand others, to foresee events or how an event might potentially develop; increased creativity; analytical thinking; and a rich inner life. But the advantages are also disadvantages. Having an analytical mind and the ability to foresee consequences makes it difficult to be in the moment and to enjoy the here and now. Having a rich inner life isolates me sometimes from the "outside" world, so I need to consciously step out of it and focus my awareness on the "external." In general, it feels like nothing is easy, everything is an object of analysis, and sometimes I think endlessly about meaning and consequence. Every beginning is a reason to think about the end.

If I had the choice to be highly sensitive or not, I think I would choose not be highly sensitive. There are many great things connected to being an HSP, as I said, but sometimes it just feels like torture. I am now in the process of accepting who I am and focusing on the advantages of this trait, and I hope I will get to a place of full acceptance soon. However, I feel like less ruminating about the ones I choose to be with would lead to a more fulfilling personal life. I could have spent much more time just living an ordinary life, instead of being almost forty years old and not really being settled. For a very long time, I felt like a terminally single person, because having close relationships was just too difficult, constantly thinking and feeling. As part of the process of accepting myself as an HSP, I finally see that this is not necessarily the only way and that with a certain focus, relationships are possible.

What are the particular difficulties of being a highly sensitive man in our society?

If I wasn't highly sensitive, I probably wouldn't be so creative and perhaps even not so successful in my career, but I think I would have a more fulfilling personal life. For example, in the current world of gay relationships, where almost every contact starts very quickly with sexual intercourse, I feel I am just out of the game, because I cannot do one-night stands. Also, I feel that many gay men have so-called "open relationships" with their partners, and that's something that doesn't work for me, as I would not be able to handle all the stimulation that would come from not being able to focus on one person and feeling the full emotional support that I need.

Also, in work situations, where group work is very much promoted, I am intimidated by environments where many people are competing with each other for who gets more attention or who will contribute more. It also takes much more time for me to respond to questions or tasks in group environments. Before I have made up my mind, others have said what they're thinking already and therefore decisions are often made quickly. If I want to express myself, I often need to fight hard for the group's attention, which is exhausting.

How does your high sensitivity impact on your relationships with other men?

This is a rather complex area. Generally speaking, I think for many years my sensitivity had influenced my friendships and relationships with other men negatively, in the sense that very often I did not maintain them or start them, because I felt inferior and was simply afraid of those friendships or relationships. The inability to deal with men in romantic relationships is probably why, at the age of thirty-seven, I have had only one serious relationship. That ended five years ago, and I'm still single.

But I have worked a lot on this, and it feels like things are improving. I have a growing sense that being highly sensitive can actually be an advantage to all types of relationships—whether with men or with women—because the quality of a relationship depends on the interaction of two people, and not on their gender identity. This approach has brought many interesting people into my life who seem to appreciate me in my complexity and accept me as I am. That, in turn, helps me to accept myself as I am, here and now, as a complex person, and not think of myself as a flawed person. I must admit that this is a relatively new feeling for me. The feeling of being accepted as a highly sensitive man by other men came when I started to realize my own worth, independent of whether others approve of me or not. Previously, I think I was afraid men would disapprove of me. I think that was not always grounded in actual experiences or facts, but more in my own fear.

When it comes to sexual or romantic encounters with other men, the biggest influence of my high sensitivity is that in order to enjoy sex with someone, I need to feel close to them and must have the feeling that we get along in other areas, too. That basically rules out having purely sexual encounters or having sex just for the fun of it. I have tried many times to "unlearn" this, but with no success. What seemed to work, at least initially, was numbing my senses with alcohol. But in the end, that only led to risky behavior, no real pleasure, and emotional difficulties afterwards, so I stopped doing that. I also had to learn to express my own needs and desires and not only focus on satisfying my partner's needs.

How does your high sensitivity impact on your relationships with women?

I have always felt more comfortable with women around, and I have been much better at starting and maintaining friendships with women. I think that's because they are generally more sensitive, or maybe just better at being open about their feelings and emotions. So it has been easier to feel "myself" in the presence of women because I didn't have to pretend or hide the sensitive part of me, but could let it show. Therefore, it is much easier for me to feel close to women. However, in close friendships or relationships, I have to make sure that I maintain certain boundaries and retain a stable sense of self, particularly with women, as I tend to feel closer to them.

What are the advantages and the disadvantages of being highly sensitive at work?

Generally, I love my job and find pleasure in it, but it's also challenging, as I get easily overstimulated. It happens on a day-to-day basis. When I'm part of a group discussion, it is very difficult for me to listen to everyone talking and to process all the stimulation coming my way. Coming up with my suggestions takes time, because I need to process the input first. When I travel for business, this often means spending up to eighteen hours a day with other people— meetings, social events, and so on. I find this so draining that I usually need at least one day on my own to recover afterwards. My job allows me a lot of flexibility, such as working from home, which suits me best. So it is a paradox: I love working with others, but at the same time, I find it challenging and draining.

I think I am good at analyzing and collecting huge amounts of data and then creating new conclusions based on that. I also think that I have good social skills and a lot of empathy, which is helpful working with others in my field.

What's your advice for other highly sensitive men?

Find a good therapist who understands you and who knows what high sensitivity is, because they will guide you in the right direction. With their support, work on your self-acceptance, as this is the only way to be happy—being happy with who you are. I have been diagnosed wrongly so many times and have been treated for depression and anxiety, while no one ever told me that what I'm going through is an inherited part of my personality that I need to accept, not a disorder that needs fighting.

The biggest lesson that I have learned is that I will not get rid of my sensitivity, but that I can learn to direct it in healthier ways and perhaps can also use it to my or others' benefit.

Strategies to Deal With Overstimulation and Intense Emotions: Mindfulness and Acceptance

NOW THAT YOU HAVE LEARNED a lot about the importance of emotional regulation for highly sensitive people and have started practicing these first exercises, I'm now going to give you some more strategies to help you get better at self-soothing when you're dealing with overstimulation and strong emotions. You're going to learn about mindfulness and how mindfulness and acceptance can help you deal with these intense feelings. Then, in the next chapter, I'm going to teach you some useful exercises to help you consciously relax your body, as well as introduce you to imagery exercises because consciously generated mental imagery and visualization can also help us to change and positively influence our feelings and their intensity.

Despite the fact that mindfulness and acceptance, relaxation, and imagery exercises are all different processes, like different tools in a toolbox, they are all examples of "emotional tools." This means that they are strategies that you can reach for when you're feeling overstimulated or emotionally overaroused. Regularly practicing and using these techniques will help you get better at calming yourself more quickly and recentering yourself in those moments in which you don't know whether you're coming or going or when you feel that you can't think straight because you're feeling overwhelmed by too much stimulation.

Research into emotions has shown that different areas of the brain are responsible for cognition and emotions. The emotional centers of the brain, often collectively called the limbic system, are, from an evolutionary perspective, significantly older than the cognitive centers of the brain, such as the prefrontal cortex. These cognitive centers are responsible for things like situational action control, alertness, thoughts, and the regulation of emotional processes. And both areas of the brain exist in a reciprocal relationship with the other, meaning that our thoughts influence our feelings and vice versa.

Lammers wrote, "The cognitive functions of the PFC [prefrontal cortex] allow human beings to distance themselves from the influence of their immediate emotions and thus achieve freedom of action. We call this emotional regulation."[1]

As long as the intensity of our emotional arousal remains in the lower to middle range, then the prefrontal cortex is pretty good at controlling our feelings and we can use tools such as increased mindfulness and forming alternative thoughts to calm ourselves down and, in turn, reduce the intensity of our emotions ("I can tolerate this situation, even though I feel very emotional in this moment"). Problems arise, however, when our emotional arousal reaches a high level, because then the more primal, emotional areas of the brain begin to impede the cognitive areas and temporarily shut off their functioning until our emotional arousal drops back down to the medium or lower range again.

Lammers also notes, "For the person being affected, the inhibition of the cortical structures of the PFC and the hippocampus leads to chaotic thoughts, confusion, and memory problems. When one experiences very intense emotions of fear, anger, rage, and high emotional tension, then this leads to an inhibited functioning of the PFC. This reduced cognitive performance affects the regulation of emotions, which, in turn, become even more intense."[2]

This explains why we find it so difficult to think clearly in moments of emotional arousal. It is in precisely these moments that we need to be able to fall back on simpler strategies that don't rely on as much cognitive effort or, more simply put, as much thinking. These simple strategies might include concrete behavioral changes, like leaving or changing a given situation or using strategies to consciously relax our bodies, to become more mindful or more accepting. Once we have managed to self-sooth using one or more of these strategies and our emotional arousal levels have dropped, we are then able to think clearly again and are better able to use those areas of the brain that are responsible for complex cognitive performance to, for instance, begin to form alternative thoughts.

This reminds me of a young highly sensitive client of mine who became so anxious when he had to do written exams at his university that he found it impossible to think straight. The strategy he developed to deal with this was simply to ask for a toilet break so that he could leave the examination room for a few minutes. On his way to the bathroom, he then had the space to calm himself down. He was able to take some deep breaths and to relax his muscles, and this brief "change of scene" helped him to concentrate and to better answer the questions when he was back in the examination room. He was suddenly able to think clearly and find the answers to questions that had stumped him moments before.

Of course, not every highly sensitive man is in a constant state of physical, cognitive, and emotional arousal. But I do think that it's important that you're aware of this very simplified illustration of how these neurobiological processes work. This knowledge helps us to understand how emotional regulation functions and why distracting our attention, in the form of mindfulness and physical relaxation, is

so important and why it should not be underestimated as a strategy
for dealing with overstimulation and intense feelings.

Mindfulness

Mindfulness is a term that has received a lot of attention over the past
few years and is used in numerous different contexts. You can "be
mindful," "live mindfully," "walk mindfully," "eat mindfully," have
"mindful sex," and "mindfully raise your children." There doesn't
seem to be any area of our lives for which countless books, magazines, and lifestyle gurus haven't suggested that we couldn't live
more mindfully. But if you are able to ignore this taint of new age
self-optimization and remain open to mindfulness, then you will
discover that it is, in fact, a genuinely good thing for our psychological and physical health. And there are numerous scientific studies
to back this up.[3] It was the American professor of molecular biology
Jon Kabat-Zinn who made the first significant steps to introduce
the originally Buddhist concept of mindfulness into Western psychotherapy when he developed his eight-week-long Mindfulness-
Based Stress Reduction course in 1979. In these courses, which have
since become hugely popular worldwide, course participants practice numerous mindfulness and meditation techniques that have
proven to be extremely effective in the treatment of depression,
chronic pain, and anxiety. The new wave of cognitive behavioral
therapies, mentioned in earlier chapters, also make extensive use of
the concept of mindfulness.

The term *mindfulness* has its roots in Buddhism and is a central
tenet in all of the schools of Buddhism that have developed over the
past 2,500 years. Originally, *mindfulness* was the translation of the
word *sati*, which means "to remember" and refers to our consciousness of the present moment. "[Mindfulness] is used in Buddhist texts
to refer to the conscious awareness that accompanies every thought
and every action."[4]

When I practice mindfulness with my highly sensitive clients, I often refer to it as "training our attention" or as "consciously directing" our attention. We try to understand what it means to embrace this and simultaneously try to develop an attitude of compassion toward ourselves and other people. Like the beam of a flashlight, we can consciously direct our attention to our *internal processes*—our feelings, thoughts, and physical sensations—and observe them without becoming "unmindful" and immediately "at one" with them or automatically reacting by behaving in a certain way. It is thus about taking on the role of the observer, as you would when you meditate. Thoughts, feelings, and physical sensations are observed as if one were sitting in a movie theater and watching them on the big screen. The goal is to not completely lose yourself in the film's plot and to keep reminding yourself that you are sitting in a theater on a seat, watching a film.

But we can also turn the beam of our flashlight onto *external processes*, that is to say, to everything that we see, hear, smell, taste, and feel through our five senses. In this case, we're trying to remain in the role of the observer without losing contact with the here and now. We don't want to get tangled up in our thoughts about what we are perceiving, or, if we do, we want to quickly register that we're doing this. An example of this might be very consciously eating a meal while being conscious of all of our senses and internal judgments in the form of thoughts ("This dish tastes great," "This is too salty," "I don't like asparagus," etc.). The art of this is remaining mindful and not becoming lost in one's thoughts, feelings, perceptions, and internal storytelling, not drifting off. And if we do drift off, that's not a problem. We should just become aware that this is happening and then bring our attention back (to the meal, for example). This back and forth between distraction and conscious attention is what is important here. It is *not* about not having any thoughts or not getting distracted.

Dr. Jan Chozen Bays, an experienced Zen Buddhist meditation teacher and a pediatrician, defines mindfulness in the following terms: "Mindfulness is deliberately paying full attention to what is happening around you—in your body, heart, and mind. Mindfulness is awareness without criticism or judgment."[5]

So practicing mindfulness isn't about never having any judgmental thoughts again. It is about recognizing that I have had a judgmental thought, which I can free myself from by recognizing the thought and then consciously turning my attention away from the thought. The opposite of this would be to "unmindfully" lose yourself in the thought, thus losing contact with the moment.

If I confront the present moment mindfully, then I hear the rain drumming on the roof; I hear a blackbird and two magpies singing (or cawing, in the case of the magpies); I feel the cool and damp autumnal air on my skin through the open window; I see the green and orange leaves hanging on the trees; I feel the chair and the cushion that I am sitting on; I notice that my feet are cold, and I perceive the hard wooden floor beneath the soles of my feet; I notice my clothing touching my skin, particularly beneath my arms and on my thighs; I feel my fingertips and palms on the warm keyboard of my laptop; and I notice that I'm hungry, and I observe my thought: "I'm hungry!"

What this example shows is how easy it is to practice mindfulness. You can do it anywhere and in any moment, even now as you're reading these lines. What can you see, smell, feel, taste, hear? How does your body feel? What do you feel? What thoughts are going through your head?

Why Mindfulness Can Help with Overstimulation and Strong Feelings

Why is mindfulness a valuable strategy for highly sensitive people when dealing with overstimulation and intense emotions? If you can learn to become more mindful, then you will change the relationship you have to your thoughts, feelings, physical sensations, and to the present moment. You will start to perceive things without distorting them through your own thoughts and judgments. You will observe and watch what you are experiencing, instead of seeing the world *through* what you are experiencing. This can lead to a valuable state of inner tranquility, clarity, and alertness. Mindfulness is thus the antidote to being on autopilot—something that we often do as we go through our daily lives—or the feeling of being so in our thoughts that we are no longer really able to perceive our surroundings and our own bodies.

If we imagine that our feelings, thoughts, and physical sensations are the water in a lake, then when we are practicing mindfulness, we are trying to watch the water from the shore rather than swimming in the water and looking back at the shore. This is particularly important when we feel very strong feelings, such as anger, excitement, or loneliness, or when we have lots of thoughts going through our heads. In these situations, we often begin to brood and risk losing ourselves in these thoughts and losing contact with the reality of the moment. Often our thoughts and judgments ("I did that right/wrong/well/badly," etc.) stoke our emotional fire, particularly when we no longer have the necessary distance from our thoughts and have long since become enmeshed in them. We can use mindfulness to help us build up more observational distance from our feelings and thoughts and through this become less defined and automatically dominated by them. This, in turn, can give us a sense of inner calm and confidence because we notice that thoughts and feelings are constantly coming and going, but we don't always need to surrender to them.

I often compare the human psyche to a radio station and consider thoughts as the songs that the station plays twenty-four hours a day. We don't love all of the songs, and sometimes it plays repeats of songs that we don't particularly like. But it can be useful to recognize that this is just the way this radio station works, that it is its job to play one song after the other. We can't change that. And the station is never going to not play any songs. But what we can change is learning not to give the song we don't like any more attention than we have to, to give it no more attention than we would give to any other song that the radio is playing. At the end of the day, it is only one song among many, and at some point even this awful song is going to stop playing. If we can do this, then we are going to find this song less annoying and it's going to seem less important, meaning that we're going to get better at tolerating it.

In this way, mindfulness can act like an anchor for highly sensitive people. You can learn to throw it out when your internal sea becomes particularly stormy and it seems impossible to form alternative or supportive thoughts to calm yourself down or give yourself strength. It is thus an emotional regulation strategy, similar to physical relaxation, that pays off particularly when you are feeling overwhelmed or particularly emotional. So mindfulness and relaxation function like a first-aid kit. Once you have successfully deployed them, you will then be in a position to use more cognitive strategies.

Structured Mindfulness Exercises

There are many different ways to learn and practice mindfulness. Alongside mindfulness courses, which are now offered in the most far-flung places, mindfulness is also taught as part of many yoga and meditation courses. Other sources of information about it include numerous books and websites. Taking part in an eight-week Mindfulness-Based Stress Reduction course offers a good introduction and can really help to reduce tension, stress, and pressure.

Aside from taking part in an actual course, there are also other ways to practice mindfulness in our everyday lives. We can, as it were, *formally* make time for mindfulness exercises and consciously integrate them into our daily routines by, for instance, taking a few minutes out of every evening to sit on a chair or meditation cushion and practice mindfulness. Or we can build mindfulness into our lives in a more *informal* way by living our lives more mindfully, rather than practicing specific exercises at a specific time. For instance, we can consciously pay attention to the food we eat, to the armchair we're sitting in, or to what we can hear when we walk down the street, instead of getting lost in thoughts and not even being aware of the street around us. A more informal exercise might be, for instance, mindfully noticing the feeling of water on our skin when we're in the shower in the morning, listening to the hiss of water spraying from the showerhead, smelling and feeling the shower gel, perceiving the way our muscles contract, focusing our attention on all of our senses. And doing this, for instance, instead of planning the day ahead—actually experiencing what we are actually doing, namely, showering. Generally, it is most fruitful to integrate mindfulness into our lives in both formal *and* informal ways.

On the following pages, you will find a range of mindfulness exercises that I have used over the course of my psychotherapeutic career. They are relatively simple exercises that are going to offer you an easy introduction to becoming more mindful in your life. I would suggest, for the first six or eight weeks, that you start by introducing a period of between five and twenty minutes daily dedicated to structured mindfulness exercises. If after completing this first phrase you want to learn more about mindfulness and deepen your practice, then I would highly recommend joining a meditation group or a weekly mindfulness course.

When you are practicing these exercises, it is important that you don't fall prey to perfectionist thinking and don't expect to free yourself from all thoughts or to achieve a particular state of consciousness or perfect inner calm. It's much more about contemplating your experience and witnessing what is going on in the present moment with compassion and clarity. The more that you practice mindfulness, the easier it will get and the better you will become at using it as an aid in moments of overstimulation and when you are experiencing strong feelings. It will also improve your ability to quickly register when you are slipping into feeling overstimulated.

If you find it uncomfortable doing the exercises with closed eyes, then just leave them open. In rare cases, some people feel anxious when they're doing mindfulness exercises because they suddenly become very conscious of their thoughts, feelings, and bodily sensations. If this is something that you experience, then just open your eyes and end the exercise, center yourself by becoming conscious of your senses in the here and now, and try again at a later point in time, perhaps starting with your eyes open to reduce the intensity of the exercise.

Mindful Listening

- Sit on a chair or on a meditation cushion. Make sure that you're sitting comfortably. If not, change your sitting position until you are comfortable. Try to sit up straight without too much tension in your body.
- Drop your head a little and focus on a point on the floor in front of you. Let your focus become blurred and soft or close your eyes, if you're comfortable doing so.
- Turn your attention to all of the sounds that you can hear in this moment. Even if you thought, at the beginning of the exercise, that your surroundings were quiet, you will now begin to notice that you are hearing more and more the longer that you pay attention.
- Silently list to yourself all of the things that you can hear in this moment: for instance, "Footsteps, the distant roar of traffic, the ticking of a clock, the hissing of the radiators, the neighbors' music . . ."
- Whenever the sounds spark thoughts or images, or whenever you become lost in thoughts or judgments ("Why do my neighbors always play their music so loud?"), try to consciously bring your attention back to the sounds. Keep consciously bringing your attention back to the sounds as often as possible.

- When you are ready, gently open your eyes at your own pace or let your focus sharpen again. Stretch and consciously bring your attention back into the room.

This exercise is a great introduction to mindfulness, and you can practice it for as long as you want, though generally you should be aiming to practice it for at least five minutes. It shows us that we can use all of our five senses and that we can keep consciously redirecting our attention back to them. In doing so, we are consciously releasing ourselves from our thoughts and feelings. This is also a great exercise to use informally, be it in the office, on the bus, or at the supermarket checkout counter. In these moments, we can try to detach ourselves from our judgments about the sounds that we hear so that we can better tolerate them.

Developing a More Mindful Contact with Your Surroundings

- Sit on a chair or on a meditation cushion. Make sure that you're sitting comfortably. If not, change your sitting position until you are comfortable. Try to sit up straight without too much tension in your body.
- Drop your head a little and focus on a point on the floor in front of you. Let your focus become blurred and soft or close your eyes, if you're comfortable doing so.
- Consciously turn your attention to the parts of your body that are making contact with your surroundings and with the floor. Feel the soles of your feet on the floor, feel where your thighs, your buttocks, and your back are in contact with the chair. Let your attention wander to other parts of your body that are touching other things, like your hands touching each other or touching your thighs. Notice how your skin feels when it's touching your clothing and when

it's touching nothing: What does the difference feel like?
Pause briefly at each of these places of contact: How does
this contact feel in each of these areas of your body? Warm?
Hard? Cold? Which physical sensations do you notice?

- If your thoughts drift or you get lost in your thoughts, then
that's not a problem. What's important is that you return
to these areas where your body is making contact with its
environment. Repeat this process, noticing each time that
your thoughts drift off and bringing your attention back to
these contact points, feeling again how these areas of your
body feel. Does the material feel scratchy on your skin?
Does it itch, prickle, or sting these parts of your body? Try
to accept these physical sensations for what they are, without evaluating them as good, bad, pleasant, or unpleasant.
- When you are ready, gently open your eyes at your own
pace or let your focus sharpen again. Stretch and consciously bring your attention back into the room.

This exercise also uses one of our five senses to train our attention. I can recall a highly sensitive client whom I worked with who
used this exercise during team meetings at work, where he often felt
overstimulated and uncomfortable. There were numerous unspoken
conflicts in his team, which he was very aware of, and during these
meetings there were lots of people talking at once. By mindfully focusing on the perception of these contact points between his body
and the chair, the floor, the table, or his water glass, he found it easier
to calm himself down in these meetings and not to stay stuck in a
state of overstimulation. The more often that he practiced this exercise, the better he became at redirecting his attention. This allowed
him to get much better at tolerating overstimulating situations, such
as team meetings, making them much more bearable.

The next exercises build on the last two. They should help train
you to redirect your attention inward so that you learn to observe
your internal processes.

Mindful Breathing

- Sit on a chair or on a meditation cushion. Make sure that you're sitting comfortably. If not, change your sitting position until you are comfortable. Try to sit up straight without too much tension in your body.
- Drop your head a little and focus on a point on the floor in front of you. Let your focus become blurred and soft or close your eyes, if you're comfortable doing so.
- Feel the areas of your body that are making contact with your surroundings and consciously keep your attention there for a few minutes. How do these contact points feel? If you lose yourself in your thoughts, notice this and return to your contact points.
- Let your attention spread out from these contact points to the rest of your body. What do you perceive? How does your body feel in this moment? Which physical sensations do you feel most strongly? Where in your body do you sense warmth, coolness, pressure, tightness? Which parts of your body are soft or tingly?
- Consciously turn your attention to your breathing. Notice how it feels to breathe in and how it feels to breathe out. Notice the differences in your physical sensations. Follow your breathing—through your nostrils, into your lungs, into your chest, into your belly—and notice your breath leaving your body again. You don't have to do anything and you don't have to breathe in any particular way, just observe this automatic, repeating process, feeling it and paying attention to it.
- Sense the point in your body where you can feel your breath most strongly (the nostrils, the chest, your abdominal wall, etc.) and try to keep your attention focused on this point. If you want, you can also put your hand on your belly, noticing the contact between hand and belly, focus-

ing on this contact point and observing how your hand rises and sinks with your breath.

- If your thoughts drift or you catch yourself judging your breathing ("I have to breathe more steadily!") or you lose yourself in a feeling (boredom or impatience, for instance), then notice this. Just gently bring your attention back to your breath and to the point at which you can most clearly feel your breath. Every time that you notice that you are drifting away, bring your focus back to your breath in a friendly and calm manner. Try to lose yourself more deeply in the automatic rhythm of your breathing.

- Slowly bring your attention back into the room. When you are ready, gently open your eyes at your own pace or let your focus sharpen again. Stretch and consciously bring your attention back into the room.

The next exercise combines elements of the last two exercises and will help you become better at consciously redirecting your attention to both external and internal processes. I often practice this exercise with my clients at the beginning of our sessions because it can help us to feel centered and to achieve a feeling of inner calm. This exercise is also particularly good when dealing with difficult feelings.

Being Mindfully in the Here and Now

- Sit on a chair or on a meditation cushion. Make sure that you're sitting comfortably. If not, change your sitting position until you are comfortable. Try to sit up straight without too much tension in your body.

- Drop your head a little and focus on a point on the floor in front of you. Let your focus become blurred and soft or close your eyes, if you're comfortable doing so.

- To begin with, turn your attention to the sounds that you can hear. Silently name a sound you can hear, then wait until you can hear the next sound.
- Now move from the external to the internal, turning your attention to the places that your body is touching the world around you. Notice how your body feels at these points. How would you describe these physical sensations? Try to accept them as they are in this moment.
- Moving out from these contact points, turn your attention to the rest of your body. Notice what you can perceive in your body and the different physical sensations that you can feel. When you lose yourself in thoughts, don't worry; just gently move your attention back to your body.
- Turn your attention to your breathing. Become aware of the flow of your breath and attentively follow the process of your breathing—from the nostrils through the chest to your belly. Notice where you can feel your breath most strongly and keep your attention there. Don't expect to breathe in a particular way, but accept your breathing the way it is in this moment and let yourself drift into the rhythm of your breathing.
- If you notice thoughts coming up and holding your attention, then briefly label the thought (for instance, "work," "family," "worries," "judgment," "weekend," "eating," "politics," "sex," etc.) and consciously bring your attention back to your breath. Repeat this process and remain kind to yourself. It is not a problem if you drift off into thoughts, but the moment that you notice you're doing it, just label the thought and bring your attention back to your breathing.
- Turn your internal focus to your feelings by asking yourself, "How do I feel in this moment?" We will sometimes be feeling a number of feelings at the same time, or it may take a while before we can clearly put a name to our feelings ("I feel lonely/relaxed/annoyed/sad," etc.). Also observe where

this feeling is located in your body (for instance, in your stomach, in your chest, your thighs, your jaw, etc.) and which physical sensations accompany the feeling. Don't try to make the feeling become bigger than it actually is and don't try to repress it, just accept the physical sensation in the moment as it is. Observe the physical components of your feeling and consciously let the part of your body that it's located in loosen by directing your breathing there or relaxing the muscles. How does this change the physical sensation and, potentially, the intensity of the feeling? Observe this for a few minutes.

- Slowly bring your attention back into the room. When you are ready, gently open your eyes at your own pace or let your focus sharpen again. Stretch and consciously bring your attention back into the room.

Informal Mindfulness Exercises

Alongside the structured mindfulness exercises that you can practice at home, it is also helpful if you can generally become more mindful in your daily life. Doing so can help us experience our lives in a more conscious way, stop us from losing touch with the present moment, and make mindfulness something less theoretical and abstract. It also has the positive side effect of slowing down our daily lives, which is something that highly sensitive people often crave. At the end of the day, practicing mindfulness informally just means paying more attention to our five senses in our daily lives, perceiving them, becoming more aware of our thoughts, feelings, and physical sensations and, through that, learning to become better at noticing what or where the focus of our attention is and being able to redirect it.

There are many books and sources of information about practicing mindfulness in our daily lives. Because of this, I'm just going to mention a few exercises here to give you a taste of the ways that you can immediately change your daily life as a highly sensitive man by more strongly integrating mindfulness into it. It may also be the case that the following exercises also spark off some of your own ideas for bringing mindfulness into your life.

Informal Mindfulness Exercises for Daily Life

1. When you wake up in the morning, take a moment and become conscious of your breath. Consciously notice where your body makes contact with the mattress, the sheets, and the pillow. Before you get up, observe for a moment your physical sensations and your thoughts. Now focus clearly on your bedroom and become conscious of what you can see and hear.

2. Mindfully prepare your breakfast. When you are standing in the kitchen, notice the soles of your feet on the floor and become aware of your posture, the movements of your hands, and your physical sensations. When you eat something, chew it and swallow it slowly and consciously, registering how your breakfast smells, tastes, and looks.

3. When you're heading to work on the bus, the subway, the train, or in your car, notice how you are making contact with the seat and the floor. Pay attention to your breathing, your physical sensations, and the thoughts going through your mind. If you are on public transportation, look out of the window and notice the colors and forms that you can see. In your head, name the things that you can see without immediately passing judgment on them. Close your eyes, if you can do so safely, and notice the sounds around you. If you are driving a car, then notice where your body makes contact with the steering wheel and the seat and turn your attention to the visual details you can see on the road in front of you.

4. Over the course of the day, keep returning to your breath-
    ing and to your physical sensations. For a few breaths,
    really pay attention to your breathing. Is part of your body
    tense? Are you able to consciously relax it? Which other
    physical sensations can you feel?

5. Over the course of the day, keep asking yourself these ques-
    tions: How do you feel in this moment? What do you need
    when you feel like this? What emotional need is being ex-
    pressed by this feeling? What might help you to fulfill this
    need (for instance, saying something encouraging to your-
    self, opening a window, spending a little time alone,
    having a break, taking a sip of water, going to the toilet,
    etc.)? Which thoughts accompany your feelings? What ac-
    tion are you tempted to take when you feel this way?

6. When you're talking to someone, consciously turn your
    attention to that person. What can you see? What is that
    person's expression, gesture, or smell? Which thoughts,
    feelings, physical sensations, and impulses do these
    things trigger in you?

7. Perform your daily tasks mindfully, being calm and dili-
    gent, be it cleaning, eating, showering, walking, shopping,
    speaking, listening, getting dressed, tying your laces,
    combing your hair, shaving, or cooking. For a while, this
    may also mean consciously doing these activities more
    slowly than usual.

Acceptance of Feelings

The examples mentioned above represent just a few of the ways that
you as a highly sensitive man can build mindfulness into your daily
life and become better at separating yourself from strong emotions
and an excess of thoughts. You may well have noticed that acceptance is a key part of mindfulness—acceptance of how things are and

not of how we would like them to be. This means perceiving ourselves and our environment as they are, without immediately trusting the judgments we assign to them (good or bad, right or wrong, wonderful or terrible, etc.). Or at the very least, noticing that this judgment is a cognitive one. Because at the end of the day, a judgment is just a thought.

But learning to be accepting doesn't just relate to thoughts or physical sensations, or to situations that we often find ourselves in, but also to the way that we deal with unpleasant feelings. When we become better at recognizing our trains of thought and can stop immediately judging our feelings as either positive or negative, or blindly trusting them, when instead we encounter them with acceptance and, in the first instance, just acknowledge and observe them, then this starves our "emotional fire" of oxygen.

Our negative feelings are often exacerbated by our own judgments about them. We have all, for instance, felt anxious or unsure in certain situations. When we judge our feelings of uncertainty and trust the emerging negative thought ("I shouldn't feel so unsure," "What's wrong with me?" "Here I go again," "I can't deal with anything," etc.), then we often reinforce the intensity of the feeling. A new emotional state thus emerges from the original emotional state. Our negative assessment of our feeling of uncertainty could lead, for instance, to a feeling of anger, rage, or even self-hatred. Then we get tangled up in these feelings, which usually just makes things worse for us, because our emotional arousal increases, rather than decreases. But when we manage, for instance, to perceive the feeling, to accept it and mindfully observe it—like a cloud formation in the sky that constantly changes—then the intensity of the feeling is going to drop without us fueling it.

It's also going to be easier to take the next step and deal with our feelings if we ask ourselves the following questions:

· Which emotional needs lie behind my feeling?
· What do I need when I feel like this?

- How can I best deal with this emotional situation—with
  my behavior, my thoughts, my body—and at the same time
  be kind and compassionate to myself? (Do I need to dis-
  tract myself? Relax? Do I need to leave the situation? Do I
  need to express my feelings here? Or remind myself that I
  can tolerate this feeling? What else?)

There is an important point here that I want to reiterate: the acceptance of feelings is so important because feelings become
stronger the more that we judge them, try to fight them, or try to get
rid of them. An alternative approach here is "radical acceptance."
The idea behind this psychotherapeutic concept is that we don't try
to change the feeling or its quality, but rather we try to change our
relationship to the feeling. We do this not by judging the feeling, but
by observing and accepting it, by feeling it. The psychology professor,
author, and founder of acceptance and commitment therapy Steven
C. Hayes explains his approach to accepting feelings as follows:
"'Accept' comes from the Latin root 'capere' meaning 'take.' Acceptance is the act of receiving or 'taking what is offered.' Sometimes, in
English, 'accept' means 'to tolerate or resign yourself' (as in, 'I guess
I have to accept that'), and that is precisely not what is meant here.
By 'accept,' we mean something more like 'taking completely, in the
moment, without defense.'"[6]

What I particularly like about this description of acceptance is
that Hayes highlights and describes the difference between acceptance and resignation. How could you as a highly sensitive man
approach your feelings with more acceptance? What is important
here is that you take on the role of the observer, which you practiced
earlier in this chapter. This means nothing more than looking *at*
your feelings, rather than looking out *from* your feelings. This means
walking along the edge of the swimming pool instead of jumping
straight into the water. This is, of course, often a complex balancing
act—neither repressing nor ignoring the feeling, not getting caught

up in everything that you feel, but rather observing, naming, and moving on. I sometimes compare this approach to standing on a railway platform, seeing what the destination of the next train is (anger? loneliness? shame? sadness? jealousy?), and trying not to get on board. And if you notice that you got on the train by accident (which, of course, happens to all of us because no one is permanently mindful and accepting), then don't get angry, but treat yourself in a friendly and understanding way (which in itself is already calming) and just get off at the next stop.

So the concept of accepting our feelings doesn't mean that we have to like them or that we want to feel them. It just means accepting that we feel the way we feel in this moment. If you can free yourself from the idea that your aim in a given situation is to get rid of the unpleasant feeling as quickly as possible (be it fear, uncertainty, a sense of inferiority, or loneliness) and see instead that you simply want to change your *relationship* to this feeling, then your life as a highly sensitive man is going to get a lot easier.

We want to accept the feeling as it is and create some space between us and the feeling. When we have accepted the feeling, we can then go on to think about what we need emotionally in this situation. (Think about the last chapter and the idea that all of our feelings express an emotional need.) And then we can think about how we might best deal with this difficult and perhaps intense feeling.

Strategies for Accepting Our Feelings

- Think about which difficult feelings come up for you most often (fear, anger, a sense of inferiority, loneliness, envy, etc.) and which feelings you find most difficult to tolerate. Sometimes this might be something you've felt since your childhood. How long have you felt like this?

What reminds you of this feeling? Now think about what you usually do in order to avoid feeling this particular feeling (for instance, avoiding particular people and situations, drinking alcohol, working a lot, avoiding being alone, going out, seeking out sex, ending friendships, never saying no, etc.). What negative consequences have these avoidance tactics had in your life? Next time this feeling comes up, begin by trying to allow it to instead of fighting it, saying to yourself, "Ah! Here it is again. And there it goes again!" Accept that this feeling comes up from time to time without resigning yourself to it or letting the feeling become more intense. What changes do you notice in your life when you do this?

· Observe your feelings for one week without trying to change them and without immediately feeling that you have to react to them. Accept everything that you feel, and be conscious of your feelings without intensifying or suppressing them. Imagine yourself as a curious researcher watching them under a microscope. This isn't about feeling things in a particular way ("I want to be happy," "I want to feel relaxed," "I want to feel confident"), but rather about observing mindfully what you are feeling and confronting both the good and the bad with acceptance—as if your feelings were a shadow that followed you around over the course of the day, constantly changing.

· When you notice one of these feelings, then notice where exactly this feeling is located in your body and what physical sensations accompany it (tense muscles in your thighs, heat in your face, pressure in your belly, tension in your jaw, etc.). Consciously allow this area of your body to become relaxed and surrender to the physical sensation and the feeling being expressed there. Make some room for the physical sensation. While you're observing this sensation, you can also describe how that part of your body feels (warm, cold, tight, heavy, etc.). Try not to remain with your thoughts or the feeling itself, but just observe the physical sensation of the feeling until it dissipates.

- Remind yourself that all feelings, even the unpleasant ones, are normal and human. Every person sometimes feels this way, and no one is completely able to avoid unpleasant feelings. You are part of life and of human existence. Our ability to feel pleasant feelings goes hand in hand with our ability to feel unpleasant feelings. If we want to feel the one, we must feel the other. Sometimes it helps to consciously remind ourselves of this when we are experiencing an unpleasant feeling.

- Consciously direct your breath to that part of the body in which the feeling is currently focused. Imagine that, with every breath, you are breathing out the feeling and breathing in calm, relaxation, and confidence. Consciously relax that part of your body, letting it become soft and heavy.

- When you're feeling an unpleasant feeling or one that leaves you feeling vulnerable, then confront that feeling with compassion, attentiveness, and kindness. Imagine the person you love most in life or who is most important to you feeling the way that you feel. How would you react? What would you say to this person, and how would you try to help? Try to deal with yourself with this level of care, warmth, and compassion. You can also place your hands on the part of the body in which the feeling is located. What do you need emotionally when you feel like this? What would make you feel better in this moment? What would you like to hear in this moment from someone you like and you feel supported by?

- When you feel an unpleasant feeling, tell yourself in a warm and caring voice that you accept this feeling and that you can bear it. If you find it difficult to tell yourself this, then imagine a loved one or someone you care about saying to you, "I know that you can bear this feeling. It will pass."

· Use your humor. Name your feeling (Fear? Jealousy? Excitement?) using a voice or a tone that you find funny or that makes you laugh. You might, for instance, imagine one of your friends saying it to you, someone you find particularly funny. What did they look like when they said it? Could this situation become, in the future, an amusing story, perhaps because it's so absurd?

SUMMARY

Mindfulness, whether it's structured or informal, has many faces and there are many different opportunities for practicing it and forms in which you can practice mindfulness and integrate it into your life. I believe that mindfulness is so important for highly sensitive men because it represents an essential form of self-soothing and thus can help us deal with overstimulation and strong feelings by bringing us more clarity and calm. It costs nothing except a little bit of time and your readiness to open yourself up to it and to practice it.

This is what I really wanted to convey to you in this chapter. And I also wanted to show you how you can introduce more mindfulness into your daily life. Acceptance, even of difficult feelings, is a key part of mindfulness and helps us to change our relationship to our feelings, which, in turn, influences their quality and intensity. But this is an indirect consequence, a side effect, as it were, not the imperative. We shouldn't be saying to ourselves, "I practice mindfulness to finally get rid of these feelings!" Both mindfulness and the acceptance of feelings represent strategies to regulate our emotions that can be used when we find it difficult to "think clearly" because we are feeling tense and stressed.

Adam: "Society as a whole would benefit if men could be open about their feelings instead of burying them or expressing them through aggression."

Adam is in his mid thirties and works as a mailman. What I find really interesting about his story is how naturally he deals with his feelings and how, through his mother, he learned as a small boy that it's okay to cry and to let other people see his feelings. He also describes how he is able to deal with his high sensitivity in the workplace and in contact with other men and how he is able to be naturally self-confident when dealing with his high sensitivity.

When and how did you first notice you were highly sensitive?

A friend on Facebook first mentioned the term *highly sensitive person* to me and was convinced that I was "one of them." I began reading about it and immediately felt comfortable with the term. I then ordered many books on high sensitivity and cried reading through all of them. Reading the books, I realized that I am a highly sensitive man.

When I was a child I was more "girly" or "genderless" than other boys. I played with both boy's and girl's toys. I have always been sensitive and have never been afraid to cry when I felt the need. When I was older, I often heard friends saying to me, "Oh, you are so sensitive!" However, I didn't know about high sensitivity until I was introduced to it by my Facebook friend.

What are the advantages and the disadvantages of being highly sensitive?

I think one advantage of being highly sensitive is that I can see things from a lot of different perspectives. I feel emotions so intensely and enjoy the small details in life. So the world becomes a very colorful place. I think that is a huge advantage: to notice the details that most people miss. Being so emotional and feeling things intensely can be an advantage as well as a disadvantage because you feel not only the positive emotions so strongly but also the negative ones. Both can make you feel easily exhausted.

Other disadvantages are, in my opinion, that I tend to worry a lot about small things and I like everything to be organized and under control. I also tend to overanalyze a lot—situations, people, their facial expressions, how I think they might feel, etcetera. Linked to this is my tendency to act in front of others how I think they would like me to act. Being a people-pleaser, in other words. I think that puts a lot of pressure on me to be a certain way and therefore I have a hard time feeling relaxed in social situations. But I'm working on this, and I'm starting to see progress the more I learn to be myself and trust that I am good enough the way I am.

Looking back, what sort of messages or feedback would have been helpful to you?

My mother taught me from an early age that it was okay to cry, even as a boy. That had a huge impact on my life because I didn't feel ashamed when I cried. I was proud of being able to do so and also to let others know that it is okay to be sad or upset sometimes. Being grown up now, I'm happy with the person I am today, but if I could change one thing, I would have liked to have heard from the whole of society that there is absolutely nothing wrong with showing feelings as a boy. I think society as a whole would benefit from men being able to show their feelings openly instead of having to swallow or hide them or to express them indirectly through verbal or physical violence or aggression.

How does high sensitivity impact on your relationships with other men?

In situations where there are a lot of "manly" men, I sometimes feel emasculated. I think those men often have a very clear image of how a man should be: tough, reserved, tough talking. It can be hard to be around those men, particularly at work, and I tend to stay away from them, though at work, of course, you can't choose your colleagues. However, macho men are not my cup of tea, and I think their idea of masculinity is unhealthy.

My male friends are quite sensitive, too, and I gravitate towards them because they are humble and kind-hearted and you can have a deep conversation with them about anything—from the smallest things to the biggest questions. So those men are more my thing. As I get older, I tend to spend my time with men who are more similar in their sensitivity.

How does high sensitivity impact on your relationships with women?

Sometimes I worry that my high sensitivity might scare away the woman I am in a relationship with. I sometimes get so exhausted by my feelings and my people-pleasing behavior when I'm with someone that I either have to lie down and rest, or cry. This does not make me feel ashamed, but I do start feeling scared that I will lose her as she might think that I'm "too difficult" to be with. I also worry a lot. Does she love me? Will she leave me? What if this happens? What if that happens? However, my current girlfriend is very sensitive, too, and therefore accepting of this. I also really easily notice my girlfriend's facial expressions, moods, and other signals she's sending. I am also very tender and gentle, can get the person I am with to open up, and can form a strong emotional bond with that person. I tend to give a lot in my romantic relationships, sometimes too much.

What's your advice for other highly sensitive men?

Read books about the subject. Accept who you are and learn more about your strengths and weaknesses. I think it is most important to learn some tools for handling situations you struggle with in everyday life. Don't be afraid to tell people if something bothers you, like loud noise. Hopefully, people are understanding and respect your sensitivity. And do what you feel is best for your body. For example, I have started using earplugs at work. Although no one else does it, as they do not seem to mind the noise, I wear them every day.

I also would suggest shutting out things in life that drain your energy. For example, I have stopped watching news programs and have also stopped reading newspapers, since I find them too negative and too draining.

Maybe also talk to or hang out with other people who are highly sensitive, both men and women. If you cannot meet others in person, I think internet forums are great for sharing experiences and thoughts with other highly sensitive people.

Another very important thing is to give yourself the time to rest. If occasionally you need to stay in bed for half a day, do it. If you need to take time out from the rest of the world, take it. You don't have to say yes to everything or everyone all the time. Recharge your batteries and don't push yourself too hard.

And finally, accept that there is nothing wrong with you. You're just different than the majority of people. Use the gifts and advantages that come with your high sensitivity.

CHAPTER 7

Strategies to Deal With Overstimulation and Intense Emotions: Relaxation and Imagery Exercises

*I*N THE LAST CHAPTER, WE learned about how we can use mindfulness and the acceptance of feelings to get better at self-soothing and to regulate our emotions. In this chapter, I want to introduce you to two other strategies that you can also use when you feel overwhelmed by too many stimuli or intense feelings: physical relaxation and imagery exercises.

In mindfulness, the key focus is awareness and observing our inner and outer processes in an accepting way. This stops us immediately from "becoming one" with our thoughts and feelings. This often leads to a state of inner calm, clarity, and relaxation, although this isn't our main aim when we're practicing mindfulness. The relaxation, clarity, and calm we achieve are instead side-effects of practicing mindfulness. In the case of conscious physical relaxation, however, achieving a state of physical and emotional calm *is* our concrete aim. Here we are not trying to learn to observe our feelings mindfully and accept them as they are, but rather deliberately trying to get ourselves into a state of physical relaxation so that we feel emotionally calmer.

You may remember that I talked about the connection between thoughts, feelings, behavior, and physical sensations. It is exactly this connection that we are using in physical relaxation and imagery exercises because our feelings and thoughts influence our body and our behavior. Whether we're feeling happy, anxious, annoyed, or stressed, these feelings are always accompanied by physical sensations, such as tension or relaxation in the body. But we can also flip this around and use our behavior and our bodies to influence and change our feelings. If you've ever tired yourself out at the gym, got a massage, or had a hot shower, bath, or sauna after a long day at work, it's highly likely that you felt more relaxed after these activities. A relaxed body leads to relaxed feelings. A tense body leads to tense feelings. When you feel tense and stressed, this will be expressed through your body, and we can use focused physical relaxation to deal with these stressful sensations.

Getting a massage or taking a bath are the kinds of behaviors that can help us relax and thus achieve a state of calm. But, of course, there are many situations in our everyday life in which we can't just say "Okay, I'm taking a bath now" or "I'm going for a walk." In these situations, we need to use relaxation techniques. It is these sorts of practical relaxation strategies that I want to introduce you to in this chapter.

I then want to show you how you can use your imagination and consciously visualize images to reduce your level of arousal and create feelings of relaxation, calm, and safety. The fact that images we create in our minds can influence us and how we feel will also probably be something that you're familiar with. Imagine in detail being stuck in an elevator, filling out your tax return, or being criticized by your boss in a work meeting; I bet these scenarios will generate unpleasant feelings. If, on the other hand, I ask you to recall the last vacation you really enjoyed, to imagine lying in the arms of someone you love, or to recall one of your favorite places from your childhood, then these images will likely generate completely different feelings in you. My point here is that we can positively use the power of our imaginations, our ability to consciously form images of places, people, animals, or memories in our heads. And you can learn to employ this technique when you are feeling overstimulated, stressed, or emotionally overwhelmed.

When we're dealing with the regulation of our feelings, it's good to be flexible. What I mean by that is that it's important to have as many tools in your toolbox as possible that are then available to you when your arousal level is too high and you're longing for more calm and tranquility. Practicing imagery exercises is just one of many tools. Give it a go, and if it doesn't work for you, that's fine, just try out another tool in your toolbox.

Different situations and contexts sometimes require different reactions. Sometimes the most important thing may be to name your feelings and work out which emotional need is being expressed in them so that you can change your behavior to address that need. Sometimes it's going to be important just to be aware of the feeling, to accept it and to observe it until it disappears. A different situation altogether may require you to make a concrete change in your behavior or to use physical relaxation to calm yourself down. Another time, it may be simplest to visualize a strengthening, positive image to help soothe yourself.

Whichever one of these tools you use, the goal is always the same: in this moment of emotional tension and stimulation, you are able to look after yourself and you are learning to deal well and responsibly with your particularly delicate, highly sensitive nervous system.

Physical Relaxation

The body scan is a key component of the Jon Kabat-Zinn Mindfulness-Based Stress Reduction course that I mentioned in the last chapter. In essence, what you are learning in this exercise is to mind-

fully scan your body. In doing so, you turn your attention benevo-
lently to different areas of your body. There are now many different
variations of the body scan. The following exercise is an adaptation
of Kabat-Zinn's original version, but has been tweaked to shift the
focus away from holding one's attention on the different parts of
one's body and instead onto conscious physical relaxation.

I advise my highly sensitive clients to practice this exercise regularly, preferably two or three times a week over a period of about
six to eight weeks. You can practice this exercise sitting or lying
down, and you can keep your eyes open or closed. If you tend to fall
asleep in these sorts of situations, then I'd advise you to keep your
eyes open. As always, don't set out to do this exercise perfectly. Striv-
ing for perfection increases the pressure on yourself and leads to you
judging yourself more negatively when you don't manage to live up
to your perfect expectations (and when do we ever?). Try to take
around twenty to forty-five minutes for this exercise.

Body Scan Focused on Physical Relaxation

- Whether you're sitting or lying down, try to find a comfortable position, close your eyes (if you won't fall asleep), and
  relax. Breathe deeply in and out three times, then continue
  to breathe normally. If you are lying down, keep your arms
  down by your sides and turn your palms to face the ceiling.
  Relax your pelvis by leaving a gap between your legs. If possible, avoid putting a cushion under your head so that your
  head, neck, and spine are comfortably aligned.
- To begin with, focus your attention on any external stimuli, such as the sounds around you, and then slowly turn
  your attention inward. Notice the contact between your
  body and the floor or chair. Observe your breathing, how
  it flows through your body completely unaided, and feel
  how your chest and your abdomen lift and sink. Where do

you feel your breath most strongly? Keep your attention there for a few minutes.

- Now turn your attention to your left foot and notice all of the sensations there—in your toes, on the sole of your foot, in your heel. What can you feel there? What do you perceive in your left foot? Warmth, cold, pressure, tingling? Where does your foot make contact with the floor or your shoe? If you can't feel anything, that's also okay, but still keep your attention just on your left foot. The moment you notice your thoughts wandering, respond with kindness and then bring your attention back to your breath and to your left foot. Now, in the second step of the exercise, try to consciously relax your left foot, letting it become heavy and loose, and release any muscle tension that you feel in your foot. Imagine your foot becoming looser, wider, warmer, heavier, and rounder.

- Now turn your attention to your right foot. Go through both steps of the exercise with this foot. Start by mindfully feeling and observing the physical sensations in your right foot and hold your attention there for a while. What do you notice? If you notice that you've become lost in your thoughts, don't worry. Just bring your attention back to your breath and then to your right foot. Then move on to the second part of the exercise. Relax the muscles in your right foot as much as you can, and allow your right foot to become loose, warm, and heavy. Notice the differences you felt compared with the same exercise on the left foot.

- Now begin to direct your attention like a beam of light through the rest of your body, each time going through the same two steps. First, become mindfully aware of that part of your body, then, consciously relax it and let the muscles and skin there become relaxed. It may help that, with every breath, you consciously breathe in and out and imagine that body part relaxing even more as you breathe out.

- Go through these two steps for every part of your body: your left calf and your left shin, your left knee, your right calf and your right shin, your right knee , . . . your left thigh, your right thigh , . . . your buttocks, your pelvic floor, your hips , . . . your belly, your chest, your left shoulder, your left upper arm, your left elbow, your left lower arm, your left hand, your left fingers and fingertips, your right upper arm, your right elbow, your right lower arm, your right hand, your right fingers and fingertips , . . . your lower back, your upper back , . . . your throat and your neck , . . . the muscles of your face, your jaw, your lips, your forehead, and your crown. There is often a lot of tension in your jaw, in your lips, and between your eyebrows.
- When you have gone through your whole body, then feel your whole body consciously relaxing and the heaviness that now spreads from your head to your toes. Enjoy this feeling of physical heaviness, and allow yourself a few minutes of very conscious calm and relaxation. If you feel part of your body becoming tense, narrowed, or tight, then deliberately relax this area again. Perhaps you are able to slip even deeper into a state of relaxation with every breath. If you notice that you have lost contact with the here and now because you've become lost in thoughts or feelings, then gently bring your attention back to your physical feeling of relaxation, warmth, and heaviness.
- When you are ready, slowly open your eyes at your own pace or allow your vision to refocus. Stretch and consciously bring your attention back into the room.

After you have practiced the body scan a number of times, you will notice how your sense of your body changes and how you casually and almost automatically start using the exercise in your everyday life the moment you begin to feel overstimulated or emotionally tense. Many of my clients use a mini-version of this exercise in just one or two parts of their body the moment that they begin to feel overstimulated or stressed—whether it be during a difficult conversation, on public transportation, in a loud restaurant, or during overstimulating social occasions.

The classic physical relaxation exercise is without a doubt Edmund Jacobson's progressive muscle relaxation (PMR). Jacobson was an American doctor who researched the connection between physical health and muscle tension, and he introduced the PMR technique in the 1920s. Since then, this technique has been successfully used internationally and is part of the standard repertoire of cognitive behavioral therapy techniques. The basic principle of PMR is that we focus our attention on different parts of our body, consciously tense those muscles, and then consciously relax them. Through this interchange of tension and relaxation, we are able to achieve a particularly intensive level of physical and emotional relaxation.

Since the 1920s, different versions of the PMR exercises have been developed. I'm now going to take you through one of the shorter variations. What is important here is that you tense every muscle group for between five and seven seconds, but then relax those same muscles for between twenty and forty seconds. You will then move onto the next muscle group and switch between conscious tension and conscious relaxation. During the exercise, try to breathe normally and take around twenty to forty minutes for the whole PMR exercise. Like the body scan, you can do this exercise sitting or lying down, and it is really worth practicing this regularly over a period of about six to eight weeks.

Progressive Muscle Relaxation

- Whether you're sitting or lying down, try to find a comfortable position, close your eyes (if you won't fall asleep), and relax. Breathe deeply in and out three times, then continue to breathe normally. If you are lying down, keep your arms down by your sides and turn your palms to face the ceiling. Relax your pelvis by leaving a gap between your legs. If possible, avoid putting a cushion under your head so that your head, neck, and spine are comfortably aligned.

- To begin with, focus your attention on any external stimuli, such as the sounds around you, and then slowly turn your attention inward. Notice the contact between your body and the floor or chair. Observe your breathing, how it flows through your body completely unaided, and feel how your chest and your abdomen lift and sink. Where do you feel your breath most strongly? Keep your attention there for a few minutes.

- Now focus your attention on your right hand and tense your right hand and lower arm as hard as you can. Keep the rest of your body relaxed. Hold this tension in your right hand and lower arm for around five to seven seconds. Notice how this tension feels, hold it, hold it, and then let the tension go. Feel how the muscles in your right hand and lower arm become loose and relaxed and keep them in this state for around twenty to forty seconds. Notice the contrast between the tension and the relaxation and enjoy this difference. Now repeat the process. Again, tense your right hand and lower arm for around five to seven seconds, and then relax both for between twenty and forty seconds. Notice how this change feels and notice the tension slowly leaving your muscles. Now include your upper arm on the right side and repeat the same transition between tension and relaxation another two times. Feel how the tension spreads from your upper arm right down to your fingertips and notice your muscles relaxing more and more.

- Now leave your right hand, lower arm, and upper arm relaxed and focus your attention on the muscles in your left hand. Tense your left hand and lower arm as much as possible while relaxing the rest of your body. Hold this tension just in the left hand and lower arm for around five to seven seconds. Notice how the tension feels, hold it, hold it, and then let the tension go and let the muscles in your left hand and lower arm become relaxed for around twenty to forty seconds. Feel the contrast between tension and relaxation and enjoy this difference. Now repeat the exercise. Tense your left hand and lower arm again for around five to seven seconds, and then consciously relax them for around twenty to forty seconds. Notice how this change feels and how the tension slowly leaves your muscles. Now bring in your upper arm on the left side and repeat the same transition between tension and relaxation another two times. Feel how the tension spreads from your upper arm right down to your fingertips and notice your muscles relaxing more and more.

· Now leave your left hand, lower arm, and upper arm relaxed and focus your attention on the muscles in your face and head. You're now going to follow the same principle: tense the muscles in your head and face for five to seven seconds, hold that tension as much as you can, and then relax it for around twenty to forty seconds. What is important here is consciously noticing the difference between the tension and relaxation and really feeling how the tension flows through your muscles. Then repeat this process twice for each part of your face. That means pulling your eyebrows together, wrinkling your forehead, scrunching up your eyes and your nose, biting down on your teeth and pressing your lips together. Hold this tension and then let your face become relaxed and smooth. Feel the difference between the tension and the relaxation and notice how your face feels. Is it warm? Is it tingling? What do you notice?

· Relax the rest of your body and focus your attention on the area around your neck and shoulders. Pull your shoulders up, push your chin into your chest, and hold this tension for around five to seven seconds, then release it, letting your body relax for around twenty to forty seconds. Again, become very mindful of your physical sensations and the contrast between the tension and relaxation. Repeat this a second time.

- Now focus your attention on your chest, your back, your belly, and your buttocks. Tense the muscles in your chest, your back, and your belly, making your abdominal wall hard and tensing your buttocks. Hold this tension, hold it, and feel it as you release it and let it leave your body. Repeat this a second time and again pay attention to all of your physical sensations.
- Now concentrate on the muscles in your right thigh and lower leg and in your right foot. Tense the muscles in your right leg and curl up your toes. Very consciously notice this hardness and tension, hold it, and then let it flow out of your body. Repeat this a second time.
- Relax the rest of your body and focus your attention on your left thigh and lower leg and in your left foot. Tense the muscles in your left leg and curl up your toes. Very consciously notice this hardness and tension, hold it, and then let it flow out of your body. Repeat the process again.
- Now tense all of your body parts, from your head to your toes, and hold this tension in your whole body for around five to seven seconds. Then let this tension flow out of your body and enjoy the feeling of relaxation for about twenty to forty seconds. Repeat this a second time.
- At the end of the exercise, take a few minutes and enjoy your relaxation and your physical sensations. Focus your attention on your breathing, and when you breathe out, let in more calm, heaviness, and relaxation. Notice the differences in how your body feels compared with at the start of the exercise and make a conscious note of them. When you are ready, slowly open your eyes at your own pace or allow

your vision to refocus. Stretch and consciously bring your attention back into the room.

If you find that PMR works for you, then you can use a shorter form of the exercise in your everyday life. For instance, you might just practice it in your hands, your arms, or your legs, switching between tensing them and then relaxing them. It's easy to do this in everyday situations without anyone around you noticing what you're doing.

Both of these exercises—the body scan and PMR—are going to help you recognize more quickly when the muscles in your body are tense or when you're reacting physically to stressful and difficult situations. They can make a huge difference if you're able, in these moments, to consciously relax your body, letting your tense muscles loosen, and focus your attention on your breathing. Taking deep breaths and then focusing on mindful breathing can really be a blessing when you feel overstimulated and overwhelmed. After relaxing your body and breathing mindfully, it can often also help to consciously focus your attention on the places on your body that are making contact with the world around them—for instance, consciously sensing when standing how your feet are making contact with the street. If you find yourself in a state of overstimulation or emotional tension, these techniques can really improve your well-being in just a few minutes and can help you to calm yourself down and make the situation much more pleasant for you.

How Do You Relax?

Over the last few chapters, I've shared many exercises with you that I use in my psychotherapeutic practice and that have been a huge help to me in my work with clients over the past few years. But there is also already a deep wellspring of wisdom, knowledge, and experience in *you*. Instead of just receiving external tips and suggestions, it can be just as important and helpful to take note of those things that you already do well when dealing with your sensitive temperament and to either take more notice of these things or build on them. Sometimes it's really not that easy to hear your own voice when there are so many voices, opinions, and suggestions pouring in from the outside world. And yet you have lived with your own nervous system and your own temperament for a very long time.

So before we look at some of the ways that you can use your imagination to help calm yourself down, I want you to think about all the ways in which you already relax and self-soothe in your daily life. What helps you to calm yourself or to come down when you feel that you've been running on full steam for too long and are about to collapse under the strain of too much internal and external stimulation? The fact that you become more quickly overstimulated and overaroused than other less sensitive men because of your sensitive disposition means that you need to create more room in your life for relaxation, calm, and time out. In other words, you need more down-time than other people. This allows your nervous system to power down and makes it easier for you to process, to digest all of the stimuli and information you've taken in. It is therefore a good idea for you to consider this and even make a priority of it in the way that you plan your daily life. Because, at the end of the day, this represents a caring and responsible way of dealing with yourself.

Relaxation in Everyday Life

1. Which activities do I find relaxing? What gives me a feeling of inner calmness?

   _____

   _____

   _____

   _____

2. In which places do I feel safe and relaxed?

   _____

_____

_____

_____

3. With which people do I feel particularly good? Which people give me a sense of safety, trust, and intimacy?

_____

_____

_____

_____

4. Which memories, images, situations, people, and places from my past do I connect most strongly with a sense of calm, security, and relaxation?

_____

_____

_____

_____

5. What kinds of music or songs, objects, fabrics, and smells calm me down and give me a sense of balance?

_____

_____

_____

_____

6. In which situations in everyday life do I generally feel the most calm?

_____

_____

_____

_____

7. Are there any routines that I have in my life that soothe and calm me and that I like doing? If so, which?

_____

_____

_____

_____

8. Which person in my life most embodies inner calm and
   composure? What would this person advise me to do
   when I feel most overstimulated, stressed, or tense?

   _____

   _____

   _____

   _____

I hope that this exercise has helped you to put a name to all of
the things that already work for you in your daily life. Try to be more
mindful of these resources and to build on them by, for instance,
doing these activities more often, meeting up more often with people
who calm you and whom you like being with, or visualizing images
and memories that you associate with intimacy, calm, relaxation,
and tranquility.

Imagery Exercises

As I mentioned at the beginning of this chapter, naming and recognizing our feelings and learning about mindfulness, acceptance, and
physical relaxation are not the only ways to regulate our arousal levels and influence our feelings. We can also do this by visualizing
positive and stabilizing images in a really focused way. In life, negative images and thoughts often push us into a state of anxiety, anger,
or worry without us even noticing it's happened. We might imagine
something happening to someone we love, think about illnesses we
could get, or start thinking on a Sunday night about the hectic Mon-
day in the office that's awaiting us, and suddenly we feel stress, heat,
or tension in our bodies. We visualize images from the past or possible futures in our mind's eye and react with feelings and physical
sensations. And we often do this in a very subconscious way.

What would happen, though, if we were to use this ability to
our advantage to generate positive images that made us feel con-

tent, secure, or relaxed? A negative image from the future is no more authentic, real, or realistic than a positive image, but both have very different effects on our bodies, on our feelings, and on our mood. I believe that the strength that comes from our ability to generate positive and stabilizing images in our mind's eye and to use these for our psychological and emotional balance is both important and enriching because we can use these images to console, calm and support ourselves. If our inner landscape, our inner life, were a garden, then these sorts of images would represent the fertilizer for the plants.

The German psychoanalyst and author Luise Reddemann describes the power of imagination as follows: "All of us have a magic ingredient available to us anywhere and at any time: Our imagination. With the help of our imagination, it is possible to create an inner world of solace, support, and strength, independent from how pleasant or benevolent the world around us actually is."[1]

Reddemann has developed a number of exercises based around imagination. I want to share one with you that was inspired by an exercise she created that focuses on our inner safe place. The inner safe place is an exercise that should help you feel calm, safe, and relaxed, and it should be really enjoyable to practice. Nearly all of the clients that I have done this exercise with in a therapeutic context really like it and have gone on to use it regularly.

If at any point during the exercise you feel unwell, then just open your eyes and mindfully anchor yourself in the here and now using your five senses. It is also important that you regularly practice this technique for six to eight weeks until you've really absorbed it. If practicing it daily is unrealistic for you, then try to practice it at least two or three times a week. It is helpful to start the exercise when you're basically feeling well and are generally reasonably relaxed because it will then be easier to use it at a later date when you are feeling anxious or nervous.

Take around ten minutes for this exercise.

Safe Place Imagery

- Whether you're sitting or lying down, try to find a comfortable position, close your eyes (if you won't fall asleep), and relax. Breathe deeply in and out three times, then continue to breathe normally. If you are lying down, keep your arms down by your side and turn your palms to face the ceiling. Relax your pelvis by leaving a gap between your legs. If possible, avoid putting a cushion under your head so that your head, neck, and spine are comfortably aligned.

- To begin with, focus your attention on any external stimuli, such as the sounds around you, and then slowly turn your attention inward. Notice the contact between your body and the floor or chair. Observe your breathing, how it flows through your body completely unaided, and feel how your chest and your abdomen lift and sink. Where do you feel your breath most strongly? Keep your attention there for a few minutes.

- Now imagine a place that feels quiet, secure, and safe. This could be a real place that actually exists or a place that only exists in your imagination. There are no limits here—all that matters is that this place triggers a feeling of calm, relaxation, and safety and that you feel positive about everything that exists in this place. It might be a place from your childhood or a place from a vacation. But it could also be a cloud, a tree house, or an island. Just see what your imagination creates. If you come up with a number of places, then pick one of these. If you can't think of anywhere, don't panic; just give yourself a little more time. It is important that you are alone in this place, though animals are allowed. Some people find it difficult to imagine being away from loved ones or people who are important to them. If that's the case, then it often helps my clients to imagine that these people are not in their immediate vicinity, but that they are in the general area and can perhaps be seen or heard.

- When you have picked a place that feels calm and safe, then dive into that image and imagine yourself in that place. You can change everything in this place to your liking; you have complete control here. But make sure that everything that you can see, hear, smell, taste, and feel is pleasant and calming.

- Look around you—left and right, up and down. What can you see? Which details, colors, forms, or visual particularities do you notice? Take note of the sounds: are there noises that you particularly like that you want to hear in this place, that are pleasant and calming? What can you smell? Do you have a favorite smell that you connect with this place that you find particularly pleasant? Can you taste anything? And what can you feel? How does your skin feel? Can you sense warmth, sun, or wind on your skin? Or perhaps some kind of soft fabric on your body? How does your contact with the earth feel here? Again, if something doesn't feel pleasant here, then just change it. You have complete control.

- Really enjoy this safe place and these feelings of calm and safety. Notice if there's something missing that you need to make yourself feel completely calm. Music? Books? Food? An animal? Photos? Whatever it is, imagine that you have it and that it feels good. Consciously look around this place again and really take in all of the impressions you get. Enjoy with every breath the calm and beauty of your special place and notice how your body feels and which physical sensations you have.

- At your own pace, slowly leave, remembering that you can always come back here anytime that you need to fill up on calm, relaxation, and strength. Take a last look around and imprint everything on your mind one last time.

- When you are ready, gently open your eyes at your own pace or let your focus sharpen again. Stretch and consciously bring your attention back into the room.

There are a range of imagery exercises that can be really helpful for highly sensitive people. The inner safe place is just one of these, but it is really a very fundamental exercise that offers a great introduction to this technique. You can, of course, develop several different places, using a different one each time.

SUMMARY

Being able to consciously activate relaxation, whether through your body or through your imagination, is a really essential tool for highly sensitive men when dealing with the overarousal that comes from too much stimulation and intense feelings. You need to be able to trust that, with the help of emotional regulation techniques, you have the power (in most situations) to calm yourself and to relax. It is therefore all the more important that you try out these strategies and practice them regularly so that you can work out which of them are particularly effective for you. I really want to emphasize again how important it is for you to prioritize relaxation and time out in your life.

Arthur: "You can be an awesome man even if you don't feel you are everything a typical man should be."

Arthur is in his early thirties and has two children. He is married and works as a social worker. He describes what effect his high sensitivity has on his role as a father and highlights the importance of good self-care and of taking regular breaks. Because highly sensitive fathers feel more quickly overstimulated than less sensitive fathers when raising children, I think he's a particularly good example of how one can deal with one's temperament in a really positive way.

When and how did you first notice you were highly sensitive?

My first memory that I can relate to my sensitivity is from my childhood. I was maybe five or six years old when we visited relatives in Finland. My mom took me out for a walk along a country road. One part of the road had more intense traffic. As a big truck drove past us on the road, I suddenly felt an intense discomfort in my whole body. I remember it was not the truck itself, but the loud noise it made that affected me. Now, as an adult who knows that he is highly sensitive, I realize that this memory is the first of many in which I reacted more strongly to loud noises than other people do.

What are the advantages and the disadvantages of being highly sensitive?

Looking back on my childhood and my teenage years, it is easier for me to find disadvantages of being highly sensitive than advantages. It was never easy for me to interact with many people at the same time. In contrast to most other boys in school, I didn't like participating in rough games. That made me feel quite lonely, and I had just one or two friends at a time. Even if I never felt comfortable in groups with other boys, I tried to fit in. For example, I played on a handball team from the ages of seven to sixteen, although I felt uncomfortable on the team at times.

As I got older, I found friends that I felt comfortable with. From ages fifteen to eighteen, the group of friends I spent time with consisted mostly of girls and one guy, who later turned out to be gay. Once I had found the right type of friends, it became easier to see the advantages of being highly sensitive. I think that I can be a good listener and a person who my friends can speak to about personal matters. I find small talk less interesting, as I'm more comfortable discussing deeper matters and topics. This fact and the fact that I'm not interested in videogames or sports make it harder to relate to men who are not highly sensitive. I often feel no connection to these kinds of men, and I sometimes wonder how they perceive me.

Looking back, what sort of messages or feedback would have been helpful to you?

Don't try to fit in if it means you have to hide your sensitive side. Try to find a social context and friends that allow you to be who you are. You can be an awesome man even if you don't feel you are every-thing a typical man should be. My stepfather always encouraged me to be myself. But I wish he would have told me not to try so hard to fit in, even when I clearly was not feeling good in certain contexts.

How does your high sensitivity impact on your relationships with other men?

When a lot of men hang out together, I often feel that I don't fit in. I don't like sports or videogames, and I find it hard to get a hold of the way men communicate in groups. Sometimes this makes me feel like an outsider.

I find it much easier to relate to women. In the past, this has led to me having more female than male friends. At my church, we tend to socialize either as married couples or in separate male or female groups. I tend to skip the male groups, and when my wife and I hang out with other couples, I often find it easier to relate to the wives in-stead of their husbands. This results in me feeling outside the "male community" at church, and I guess some men find me a little odd. On a positive note, I do have deep and meaningful conversations with the few male friends that I have.

Since I was a teenager who didn't feel part of the typical mascu-line group, I also questioned my sexuality for a couple of years. I'm now happily married to a woman and no longer question my sexu-ality, but I think I did it in the past because I simply didn't fit the typical idea of what a man should be like.

How does high sensitivity impact on your relationships with women?

Since I was a small child, I have always found it easier to relate to women. At my wedding, my mom made a speech where she reflected on this. She said that she thought that it was because I want to experience deep and meaningful relationships with other people. I think she is right. But understanding this and myself has been a struggle. Over the last couple of years, I have started to appreciate the fact that I find it easier connecting emotionally to women than to men who are not highly sensitive.

What are the advantages and the disadvantages of being highly sensitive at work?

At work, I struggle most with situations in which there are a lot of people around me. For example, once a week we have a staff meeting, which is attended by eight colleagues of mine. All the stimulation in the room, like the noise and people's moods and energies, makes me feel tired very quickly. What I also find difficult in my role as a manager at work is having to have a conversation with one of my colleagues about their behavior or the mistakes they have made. In these situations, I tend to think a lot about how the other person—whose behavior I'm criticizing—is feeling.

But being highly sensitive also has advantages in my job. I think I'm good at making my clients—who are children and teenagers that often have experienced traumatic and horrible situations in their pasts—feel that I see them as individuals and that I empathize with them. My goal as a manager is to maintain a spirit of empathy among the staff and to create a good working atmosphere. I think my colleagues appreciate me as their manager because I am attentive to their moods and wishes and I value them speaking their minds. The ability to pick up on subtle signals from people helps me tremendously when it comes to dealing with clients and with my team.

Before I became a social worker, I used to be a security officer. This was a job where physical strength was rewarded and showing a softer side was not appreciated by some colleagues. Now I have found a workplace and colleagues that appreciate my sensitive side, and for the first time in my life, I can truly be myself.

What are your strategies to deal with overstimulation and being a highly sensitive father?

What I struggle most with being a highly sensitive dad of two children is overstimulation, so developing a strategy to avoid overstimulation is key. For me, getting as much sleep as possible is really important. But prioritizing sleep also means that I don't engage in other activities as much as I used to. I try to focus on my role as a parent and nothing else when I'm at home with the children. I have also learned that it is really important for me to relax after being in a potentially overstimulating situation, like going to a shopping center or spending time with a lot of other people at work or at church.

I think that I tend to be more careful than other dads. I have noticed that many other dads just let their kids play without close supervision. I try to be close to my son and at the same time give him the freedom to try most things that he finds interesting. As a highly sensitive dad, I think I notice more of my children's emotions than a dad who isn't highly sensitive. Being constantly aware of my son's emotions and his interactions with everything around him is potentially overstimulating. When I was on parental leave, I spent a lot of time with a male friend who was also on parental leave. I think my friend found it a little bit strange that I was so strict with my time planning. I felt I had to sleep or rest when my son was asleep. Resting in the middle of the day helped me relax after a few hours with my son.

What are your self-care strategies, and what lifestyle changes have you made?

The most important change I have made over the past couple of years, apart from prioritizing sleep and rest and avoiding multitasking, was to stop drinking alcohol as I realized that I reacted very sensitively to the effects of alcohol. An internal change has occurred as well as I have decided not to try to fit in to the role of how society pictures the "ideal" man. I have decided to be happy with my sensitive side and accept it. I have chosen a profession which suits my high sensitivity, and I can use the advantages it offers.

What's your advice for other highly sensitive men?

Don't try to make yourself fit in. Not in how society thinks a man should be—strong in every situation, unemotional, not being able to relate to women—nor in situations in which you feel you have to hide your sensitivity.

CHAPTER 8

Your Relationship with Yourself: How Do You Relate to Your High Sensitivity?

H OW DO YOU TREAT YOURSELF? This question might sound a bit strange at first, or perhaps you've never really thought about how you normally behave toward yourself. When we think about relationships, their shapes and their patterns, then we're usually talking about relationships with other people—partners, friends, family members, or children. But what about the only relationship that we are guaranteed to have for the whole of our lives? How do you deal with this relationship in terms of your thoughts and your behavior when, for instance, you're feeling anxious, stressed, or lonely? What is your internal reaction when your sensitive temperament suddenly makes an appearance and ruins your plans? Perhaps, for instance, because you feel quickly overstimulated or exhausted in moments in which you need stamina and inner calm or in which other less sensitive men appear more confident and more relaxed?

In these sort of situations, do you tend to put yourself down and judge your highly sensitive reaction negatively by criticizing yourself in your head ("It was always clear that I wasn't going to manage it," "I'm just not as good/masculine/popular/extroverted as the others")? Are you excessively demanding with yourself ("You're not doing enough," "I need to create/achieve/work/accomplish more," etc.)? Or do you fall into an icy, distant silence and try to ignore your emotional, overstimulated side as if it didn't exist? Whatever your internal reaction is—and it may be none of the reactions I've described here—I think it's really important that you start to observe how you react in these kinds of situations more closely as well as how you treat yourself. Because this is where your relationship with yourself and with your high sensitivity is being most clearly expressed.

Over the last few chapters. you have been introduced to and practiced a range of techniques to regulate your emotions, and I have explained why emotional regulation is particularly important for highly sensitive men, which is backed up by the scientific findings mentioned earlier in the book. In this chapter, I want to help you develop a more caring and self-compassionate *inner* relationship with yourself. Because this is also something that can reassure us. I want to show you how you can relate to yourself in a kind, respectful, and supportive way even in difficult moments and in doing so stay by your side and not abandon yourself emotionally. Imagine a friendly, reassuring protector saying, "Yes, this is a difficult feeling, a difficult moment. But do you know what? Stay calm. I'm here for you, and we're going to get through this together!"

The Effects of Having Experienced Rejection

I don't know, of course, how other people in your life have reacted to your sensitive temperament or how you would describe your relationship with yourself generally and with your high sensitivity in particular. It may be the case that you have predominately had very positive experiences and have long since learned to like the highly sensitive side of your personality. But if not for all, then certainly for many highly sensitive men, this is not the case. They sometimes struggle with their sensitivity, are ashamed of it, perceive it as something unmanly, try to hide it, and would like to just get rid of it. This was exactly the case with my highly sensitive client in London whom I talked about in the introduction.

The majority of highly sensitive men whom I interviewed while researching this book describe growing up with a feeling that they did not fit with the conventional Western masculine ideal, the masculine norm. And this feeling has often had a deep and far-reaching effect on their relationship with themselves and on their sense of self-worth. Often this feeling of being different was already apparent in childhood. Many men also describe how their attitude toward their own sensitivity, and the characteristics and behaviors connected to it, was in large part influenced by the reactions of the other people that they grew up with. Or to put it more precisely, the way that parents, siblings, friends, family members, other school-children, and teachers reacted to their sensitivity during childhood often mirrors the way that highly sensitive men react to their own sensitivity as adults.

Let's take your relationship with your father as an example. I would assume that you would find it easier to have an accepting, positive attitude to your sensitivity—and the behaviors and characteristics that go with it—if, as a highly sensitive boy, your father gave you the feeling that he loved you. If he gave you the feeling that he accepted you and was open to you crying, to you not wanting to do things that were typical for boys, to you being withdrawn in groups or asking many questions because you were already thinking about so many things at that young age. If, however, you often felt shamed, criticized, and humiliated during your childhood and youth, perhaps because your father could not accept the highly sensitive aspects of his son—perhaps because he himself didn't like his own sensitivity or interpreted his untypical, soft, and possibly introverted son as a threat to or failure of his own masculinity—then I would assume that this has left its mark on you. In this case, the external critic—here the father—often becomes the internal critic of later life. As such, we go on to react to our own sensitivity as if it were a defect, a flaw, rather than an asset. And this is simply because we grew up with the impression that our own sensitivity was not ideal or at least not wanted in a boy.

At the same time, your personal experience within your family and within your social environment is also working in tandem with all of the social expectations of what it means to be a proper boy or a proper man. Many highly sensitive men tell me that their parents dealt with their sensitivity in an accepting way, but that other kids at school teased or shamed them for being sensitive or for being different. Many of my clients have talked about being on the receiving end of verbal aggression and rejection, being called a "sissy," "wimp," "crybaby," "little girl," or "faggot."

As mentioned in the first chapter, these socialization processes begin very early in life, and, I believe, the stiff and tight masculine suit of armor that men develop in response creates an enormous amount of pressure, shame, loneliness, and emotional pain in all men, whether highly sensitive or not. I sometimes wonder if, in fact, any man actually feels deep down that he fits the masculine ideal and conventional masculine norms. At the same time, I have the impression that it is often particularly difficult for highly sensitive men and boys because they naturally exhibit characteristics and behaviors that are not always easy to reconcile with this very tight masculine armor.

The negative or critical attitude toward a completely essential part of yourself that this leads to ("Why am I so sensitive?" "I'm just too sensitive," "I wish I was as tough as everyone else," etc.) and the potentially negative experiences in life and in relationships with other people that go hand in hand with it (for instance, being shamed, sidelined, rejected, etc.), often lead to problems of self-worth among highly sensitive men. This can manifest itself in later life as difficulties in a range of different areas and situations, such as meeting new partners, being assertive in the workplace, or taking part in activities that are dominated by men or are seen as being typically masculine. These kinds of situations can be particularly challenging and difficult for highly sensitive men and, I have observed, are often, although not always, connected with a high degree of uncertainty, fear, nervousness, self-doubt, and discomfort.

I'm going to talk about the subject of self-worth in more detail in the next chapter. So let's stay with our relationship with ourselves. Let's imagine for a moment that you are able to change your internal reaction to your high sensitivity in those situations in which you are suddenly confronted with the apparent disadvantages of your high sensitivity in your everyday life. Let's imagine that, instead of becoming critical, hostile, demanding, or disregarding, you are able to be there for yourself. In other words, let's imagine that it is in precisely these situations that you became your own best friend and began to support yourself cognitively, emotionally, and through your actions and behaviors. In precisely that moment when your sensitivity annoys you the most or when you're particularly suffering because of your tendency to feel overstimulated and to respond with high emotional reactivity. Just like you would be there for a good friend or someone else you loved who was having a hard time or was dealing with emotional difficulties. When you're confronted with emotional suffering in someone like this, I bet that you don't immediately become overly critical or hostile and angrily hiss, "Just pull yourself together!" Instead, you probably try to help such people by showing compassion, putting your arm around them, supporting them, or encouraging them. Why do we so often treat ourselves so differently when we're distressed? I sometimes get the impression that we treat ourselves in a way that we wouldn't treat anyone else. (Except maybe someone we really hated . . .) Don't you also deserve protection, intimacy, compassion, and support in these moments?

But why does learning to treat yourself in an empathetic and caring way even matter? As I've been highlighting over the last three chapters, being able to regulate one's emotions well is partic-ularly important for highly sensitive people. Alongside the techniques and exercises that you've been introduced to, what is also key is your internal reaction to those characteristics that stem from your high sensitivity, such as depth of information processing, overstimulation, emotional reactivity, and sensitivity to subtle stim-uli, as well as a tendency to be introverted. The way that you talk to yourself and deal with yourself emotionally and behaviorally is ex-tremely important, particularly if you want to reduce your physical, emotional, and cognitive level of arousal and feel calmer and more centered again. We can criticize and blame ourselves, increasing the pressure on ourselves and our emotional arousal and stress, fan-ning the flames and maintaining the internalized sense of rejection we feel from our past. Or we can try to starve the fire of self-hatred of its oxygen and create a healthy relationship with ourselves through a compassionate, accepting, caring, and self-soothing at-titude toward ourselves and our temperament.

Self-Soothing and the Psychological Benefits of Self-Compassion

Numerous studies carried out by the psychology professors Kristin Neff and Paul Gilbert have shown a clear relationship between psychological health and (self-) compassion. The more compassion-ate we are to ourselves, the less we suffer from depression, anxiety, and stress.[1, 2] If we can manage to treat ourselves with respect, care, and compassion instead of becoming self-critical ("Why can't you manage this when no one else has a problem with it?"), then we will be able to calm ourselves down physically and emotionally much more quickly and will thus be able to maintain our motivation when faced with challenges and setbacks.[3] This is particularly the case in difficult situations when things are not going well and we feel, for instance, insecure, anxious, overwhelmed, or sad. Psychotherapist

and author Christine Brähler defines the term *self-compassion* as follows: "Self-compassion is the ability to recognize that one has
experienced something painful, to allow oneself to feel this, and then
to care for oneself in a compassionate way—whether mentally, emotionally, physically, or behaviorally."⁴

This is how self-compassion complements the practical exercises introduced earlier by helping us develop a compassionate *inner
attitude* to ourselves. We can learn to generate calming, tolerant, and
soothing thoughts and images, and through this, to calm ourselves,
give ourselves credit, empower ourselves, and thus stand by our own
sides in difficult situations. We can learn to be compassionate about
our high sensitivity because, as we have learned, being highly sensitive is not always easy, particularly for men.

If you can be a true protector and friend to the highly sensitive
part of yourself, instead of falling into self-criticism and rejection,
then not much can happen to him or, at the end of the day, to you
as a whole and complete person—however other people react to your
sensitivity and however overstimulated or overemotional you feel in
a particular situation.

Gilbert, the founder of compassion focused therapy, believes that
the human brain contains at least three types of central emotional
regulation systems that interact with one another and that each give
rise to a different set of emotions in us.

1. The **THREAT SYSTEM (DETECTION AND PROTECTION)** is
   aimed at registering threats as quickly as possible, choosing an appropriate reaction (fight, flight, freeze, or some
   other coping mechanism), and flooding us with emotions,
   such as anger, fear, and disgust.⁵

2. The **DRIVE SYSTEM (RESOURCE ACQUISITION AND ACHIEVE-
   MENT)** helps us to acquire resources and to follow goals,
   like sustenance, sex, comfort, friendship, status, and
   recognition. This system kicks in the moment that barri-

ers to our wishes and goals become a threat and create
anxiety and frustration or anger.[6]

3. The third emotional regulation system is called the
   **SAFENESS-CARING SYSTEM (SOOTHING, CONTENTMENT, AND
   CARING)** and is related to feelings of contentment, calm,
   and conciliation—feeling like you don't have to defend
   yourself, don't need to chase after any goals, but are able
   to feel relaxed, calm, and balanced. Gilbert uses the example of an infant who is comforted by its parents when it's
   upset. The attention and benevolence of other people also
   comforts us as adults when we're upset and gives us a feeling of security in our daily lives.[7]

When you practice self-compassion, then you are strengthening,
in a very targeted way, your safeness-caring system—a system that
every mammal carries—and you are bringing your three emotional
regulation systems back in balance and avoiding threat-focused or
reward-focused emotional states and behaviors. This allows you to
achieve a state of inner calm, security, and emotional relaxation
more quickly—exactly the thing that many highly sensitive men
often long for when they feel overstimulated or emotional.

For this reason, the development of more self-compassion represents another important emotional regulation strategy because
it strengthens our ability to calm and soothe ourselves. If, as a
highly sensitive man, you already have at your disposal a powerful
gift for empathy, why wouldn't you use this strength and give *yourself* a little compassion?

Neff believes that self-compassion consists of three essential
components:

1. Common humanity (vs. isolation)
2. Mindfulness (vs. over-identification)
3. Self-kindness (vs. self-judgment)

Neff uses the term *common humanity* to refer to the importance of consciously reminding ourselves that we are all in the same boat and that all the people in the world experience suffering in their lives, whether they're young or old, rich or poor, male or female, Christian or Muslim. Suffering is part of human existence. If you are currently going through a difficult time in your life or have recently experienced loss, rejection, or disappointment, then don't forget that you are not alone; there are other people in the world who are also experiencing the same thing, and none of us can avoid suffering and painful emotions. It connects us as people. To regularly remind ourselves of this can help us to feel less isolated and alone and to feel more of a connection with other people.

When I see clients who have been treated in a psychiatric clinic as inpatients or who have taken part in a self-help group and I ask them what they found most helpful about these experiences, they most often say that it was the feeling of "not being alone with their problems" when they were among other people and seeing that "other people felt the same as I did." I think that this is a great example of the experience of our common humanity. As a highly sensitive man, it can also be important to remind yourself in difficult moments that you are not alone. There are many men in the world who know exactly how unpleasant it is to feel overstimulated or to be shamed about their sensitivity by other people. These men share this experience with you. This is one reason why I encourage my highly sensitive clients to meet up with other highly sensitive men.

By this point in the book, you will already be really well versed in mindfulness, so I don't need to repeat here how important it is for you as a highly sensitive man.

Self-kindness refers to the ability to treat oneself with kindness, rather than with self-criticism, rejection, or excessive demands, particularly in those moments in which things are not going well. For the rest of this chapter, let's practice doing exactly that.

Being In Contact with Your Highly Sensitive Self

If you want to change your relationship with yourself and to develop a friendly, kind, and supportive attitude to your own high sensitivity, then it can be very helpful to imagine that you as a person consist of a number of sometimes contradictory parts. The idea of accepting that every person consists of different facets, different selves, different ego states, or different "schema modes"—as they are called in schema therapy—has a long tradition in many psychotherapeutic approaches.[8] Put most simply, I'm sure that you have all experienced that different people and different situations bring out different sides or parts of you or that you've been plagued by an emotional conflict because one part of you wants something while another part doesn't. Or perhaps you've experienced situations in which you suddenly felt like a little boy again or like an excited teenager, despite the fact that you're a grown man. Perhaps you also know the feeling of suddenly being attacked by an old feeling from your childhood that comes up in specific situations that resemble past situations. All of these things are examples of how differentiated the human self is and how particular experiences, messages, and important people can have a long-term influence on us. The concept of talking about parts of oneself that can describe different, sometimes contrary emotional states and behavioral impulses—as well as typical thoughts connected with these states and impulses—can help us to better understand and deal with our emotional conflicts and change the way that we handle difficult emotional states.

If we are going to use the idea of the existence of multiple parts of the self to help us answer the question of how we can better deal with our relationship to our high sensitivity, then this requires two things of us. First, that we find and cultivate a sense of compassion, caring, and warmth and that we act from this internal position when we are looking at the highly sensitive part of ourselves. Second, that we develop an image or at least a consciousness for both the compassionate and accepting part of ourselves and the highly sensitive part. If we are able to strengthen this "inner protector," who springs into action whenever our highly sensitive part feels stressed, over-stimulated, overwhelmed, or emotional and looks after this sensitive part and calms him down or strengthens him, then you will have a guardian for life. The more often you practice these exercises based around looking after yourself, the better you will become at this and the quicker you will notice when the highly sensitive part of yourself is reaching out to tell you it needs your support, reassurance, or acceptance. So let's start developing our compassion!

Developing Compassion

- Whether you're sitting or lying down, try to find a comfortable position, close your eyes (if you won't fall asleep), and relax. Breathe deeply in and out three times, then continue to breathe normally. Feel where your body is in contact with its surroundings and lay your hand lovingly and caringly over your heart. Feel the contact between your hand and your chest.
- Think of a person from your life (partner, child, friend, etc.) whom you love or at least like very much; what is important here is that you don't wish this person any suffering. If you find this difficult, you might want to think of a favorite animal.
- Now imagine that this person (or animal) is having a bad time—perhaps stressed, afraid, sad, or in some kind of emotional need. Try to imagine this person experiencing this emotion at a level that you can tolerate and that doesn't completely overwhelm you. Now imagine this person down to the very last detail—facial expression, posture, voice, appearance, clothing. . . .
- Once you have a relatively clear image, turn to this person and try to feel as much compassion, warmth, affection, and

support for this person as possible. Before you say anything to this person or express your compassion through your behavior, it is important that you generate as much compassion, warmth, and affection as possible and that you really feel this. Notice how this compassion feels.

· Really feel your desire, which is being generated by your compassion, to reduce the suffering of your loved one. Now, in your imagination, express your compassion and your desire to help, both verbally and through your actions. Perhaps there is a word or a few sentences that you want to say to this person. Notice the warm and caring tone in your voice. You can also express your compassion physically by putting your arms around the person or putting a hand on their shoulder. Keep this image in your mind for a few minutes.

· When you are ready, slowly open your eyes at your own speed. Notice again the contact between your hand and your heart. Stretch and consciously bring your attention back into the room.

The next exercise, like the last, is inspired by one of Gilbert's exercises. The aim of this exercise is to develop an image of our highly sensitive side, to offer it compassion, warmth, and affection, and to take care of it. Many of my clients find this exercise particularly effective and powerful when the person they imagine looking after is their younger highly sensitive self. This means deliberately getting in touch with your inner child and, as the grown man you are today, taking care of the highly sensitive teenager or boy who you once were. We sometimes find it easier to feel protective, compassionate, and affectionate when the recipient of these feelings is a vulnerable child.

Another potential outcome of this exercise is that you will also get more in touch with the unfulfilled emotional needs that you had as a highly sensitive boy, which were perhaps not satisfied by your parents, other guardians, or your social surroundings. In other words, it may be the case that this exercise will make it clearer to you what you actually would have needed to hear or to receive from those around you when you felt overstimulated, afraid, sidelined, or insecure in your childhood. Someone saying, "Stay calm. Take it slowly. I'm here. We'll do this together," or, "It's not easy feeling over-aroused or overstimulated. But it's also not so bad, and it happens to me too sometimes. It'll be over soon." It may be the case that sim-ply "I like it that you're very sensitive" would have been enough.

Whatever you experienced in your childhood and whatever you actually needed or wanted from your parents and those around you in relation to how you dealt with your sensitivity, you now have the power to be a good father and a good friend by developing and strengthening your own inner protector. If you are one of those men who has or had a very difficult relationship with his father, then this might also offer you a little consolation.

Developing Self-Compassion for the Highly Sensitive Part of You

- Whether you're sitting or lying down, try to find a comfort-able position, close your eyes (if you won't fall asleep), and relax. Breathe deeply in and out three times, then continue to breathe normally. Feel where your body is in contact with its surroundings and lay your hand lovingly and car-ingly over your heart. Feel the contact between your hand and your chest.
- Now, from the last exercise, imagine again the loved one (or animal) you want to help being in emotional need. Imagine this person down to the very last detail—facial ex-pression, posture, voice, appearance, clothing....
- Try again to allow as much compassion, warmth, and car-ing build in you as possible and to perceive that person

standing in front of you. Now, in a second step, try to express your compassion and your affection verbally with a warm, friendly voice, and perhaps also express your support physically or through your behavior. Notice how the person reacts to your care. How do they look? What do they say? What do they need from you to feel better? Hold onto this image for a moment.

- Now let this image of your loved one fade. Imagine now an image of your overstimulated, highly sensitive side forming. It may be the case that your highly sensitive side is accompanied by strong feelings—uncertainty, fear, sadness, or shame. It may be your young, teenage, or adult sensitive self that finds itself in need. If you find this difficult, then simply think about the last situation in which you felt that you particularly suffered because of your sensitive temperament. Try to see yourself in this situation and notice the details here—your expression, your posture, your voice, your appearance, and your clothing.

- Try to hold on to the feeling of compassion that you felt for your loved one and direct this now to your highly sensitive self, who is suffering. Feel as much compassion, warmth, affection, and caring as you possibly can.

- Notice your desire—stemming from your compassion—to reduce the suffering of your highly sensitive self. In your imagination, express your compassion and your desire to help, both verbally and through your actions. What do you want to say to your highly sensitive self? Use a caring and warm tone of voice to do this. You can also express your compassion physically by putting your arms around the image of yourself or putting a hand on his shoulder. Be there for your highly sensitive self like a loving father or a good friend and notice how your highly sensitive self reacts and what else he needs from you or would like to hear. Keep this image in your mind for a little while.

- When you are ready, slowly open your eyes at your own speed. Notice again the contact between your hand and your heart. Stretch and consciously bring your attention back into the room.

These are both good exercises to practice regularly—perhaps during the day when you have a few minutes for yourself, or maybe in the evening before you fall asleep. What is important here is that you practice this long enough that it becomes easier to activate these images and feelings inside you.

The aim of the next exercise, which also stems from Gilbert's compassion focused therapy, is to develop your compassionate self.

The Compassionate, Calming Self

- Whether you're sitting or lying down, try to find a comfortable position, close your eyes (if you won't fall asleep), and relax. Breathe deeply in and out three times, then just breathe normally. Feel where your body is in contact with its surroundings, and lay your hand lovingly and caringly over your heart. Feel the contact between your hand and your chest.
- When you have achieved a feeling of calm, imagine an image of yourself as a particularly calm, compassionate, and benevolent person. Even if you don't normally notice these characteristics in yourself in your real life, imagine how you would look if you did embody these qualities. Take notice of all of the details of your compassionate self— your expression, your gestures, your posture, your clothing. What does your voice sound like? For a few minutes, allow yourself to imagine your compassionate self in great detail.
- Now spend some time with your compassionate, calming self and enjoy his presence. What does he say to you? What

does he suggest you do? How does he express his benevolence and his accepting care of you?

- Think about what you need from your compassionate self and what you would like to hear from him. What would do you good? Express how you're doing and what you're feeling or what you're currently finding difficult in your life. How does he react? How can he support you? Allow a dialogue to develop between you and your compassionate self.

- Enjoy the calm, the caring, the support, the acceptance, and the benevolence of this situation and your contact with your compassionate self. When you notice this feeling of inner calm, warmth, and relaxation in yourself, then slowly say goodbye to him. Remember, though, that your compassionate self is always by your side and that you can always fall back on him when you need him.

- When you are ready, slowly open your eyes at your own speed. Notice again the contact between your hand and your heart. Stretch and consciously bring your attention back into the room.

The next time you feel tense or overstimulated at a party, at a noisy restaurant, or in the office, perhaps because you have to interact with a lot of people at the same time or because the situation requires you to multitask, start by mindfully noticing this. Then ask yourself what you need in this situation so that you can better tolerate it. You might, for instance, want to seek out a quiet space, close your eyes, practice some mindful breathing, and consciously relax your body. Also imagine that your inner protector, your compassionate self, is by your side to comfort you and strengthen you. What would he say to you in this moment? You might try to take on his relaxed and confident posture, his behavior, his expression, his gestures or tone of voice and try to embody these things in the real situation. This is just one example of how all of these emotional regulation strategies that you've been introduced to could be used in different combinations in a really practical way.

Some of my clients find it easier to imagine a "compassionate companion" rather than a compassionate version of themselves. This counterpart could be a fantasy figure or even a real person in your life whom you connect with a particularly high degree of compassion, caring, warmth, acceptance, and benevolence in relation to yourself. It is even possible to use a slightly altered version of a real person. For many people, it might be a teacher or mentor they once knew, a family member, or their best friend. All that matters is that this person radiates calm, acceptance, and compassion. It doesn't matter whether you prefer a compassionate self or a compassionate companion—just stick to the option that feels right for you. You may sometimes notice that these two variations begin to mix together after a while. That's fine. Just stay creative and open to making these exercises your own.

Talk to Yourself!

At the end of the day, what all of these exercises aim to offer you is the possibility of creating a more loving and supportive relationship with yourself by actively connecting with your highly sensitive side and approaching him with compassion, calm, acceptance, and support. Talk to yourself, notice what your highly sensitive self needs when he gets in touch. How can you bolster him? How can you console him or support him? When you act from an inner attitude of compassion and calm, then your highly sensitive self will have found in you a paternal or friendly protector. Combined with the techniques and exercises that you have already learned, this will help you to calm yourself more quickly and to deal better with the challenging situations that arise in daily life as a highly sensitive man. It can also help you break the spiral of self-critical thoughts that often have an impact on our self-worth.

Dialogue Between Your Inner Protector and Your Highly Sensitive Side

TIME AND DATE	ACTIVITY/ SITUATION	HIGHLY SENSITIVE SIDE *(What is the highly sensitive part of me saying in this situation? What does he feel and think? How does he want to act?)*	EMOTIONAL AND PHYSICAL NEEDS *(What would do the highly sensitive part of me good—physically, emotionally, and cognitively? What does he need? What emotional needs are being expressed in how he feels?)*	INNER PROTECTOR *(What is my inner protector's answer? How can he react to the emotional needs of my highly sensitive side? How can he best look after my highly sensitive side?)*

On a regular basis over the course of the day, and particularly in situations that are very challenging for highly sensitive men, you can ask your highly sensitive side, "What do you feel in this moment? How are you doing?" After your sensitive side has answered, you can then ask him, "What do you need in this moment emotionally? How can I help you?" Perhaps your highly sensitive side needs your encouragement or to hear that he just needs to hold out for a little longer because the challenging situation is almost over. Or maybe he wants to be praised or reassured. Of course, it might be the case that he says to you, "Get me out of this situation! I really don't feel well!" If that's the case, then you also need to react here in a considered and responsible way.

The next and final exercise in this chapter is a dialogue between your highly sensitive side and your inner protector, based on either your compassionate companion or your compassionate self. This should help you to get better at talking to yourself on a regular basis and to strengthen the contact and communication between these two parts of yourself.

You can also practice this exercise in the form of a journal over several days and weeks, writing down situations that have occurred on each day that you found particularly challenging. But, of course, because high sensitivity is not just a disadvantage but can also be enriching and advantageous in many situations, it is worth also recording positive situations here.

SUMMARY

This way of talking to yourself and developing an inner protector for your highly sensitive side is probably going to feel slightly strange to begin with. But if you are able to make this change and to practice it, then the way you feel in your sensitive skin is going to improve substantially.

In many ways, becoming a friend to yourself and treating your high sensitivity with benevolence and acceptance is really the heart of this book. For one thing, all of the strategies introduced in this book will work best if you are able to act from this friendly and compassionate inner attitude when you are looking at yourself. To add to this, it will help you challenge those earlier emotional injuries that you likely experienced at the hands of other people who perhaps said you were "too sensitive." Dealing with yourself can, of course, sometimes involve being strict and focused, but it should never mean rejection, shame, punishment, or extreme criticism.

The themes of our next chapter—self-worth and self-care—are also strongly connected to the way that we deal with ourselves and to our attitude to our high sensitivity.

Michael: "Take your needs seriously."

Michael is in his early forties and works in a health and education context. He highlights the importance of acknowledging your temperament when choosing which career to follow and describes how difficult it is to be a man who doesn't fit the "extroverted, daredevil" ideal.

When and how did you first notice you were highly sensitive?

It was in 2015 that I first heard about high sensitivity as a phenomenon and as the subject of scientific studies. My girlfriend told me about a radio program she'd heard about high sensitivity. Shortly afterwards, a friend of ours lent us a book about it. Finding out that being a highly sensitive man was a thing and that it was being researched was a huge relief to me. There'd been so many moments in my life when I'd felt like I was different from the norm, and suddenly there was a plausible explanation. The fact that I behaved differently had been legitimized. At the same time, the whole thing seems a bit old hat to me, because I immediately felt like, "Yeah, of course it's like that, of course this is a thing." I can remember really clearly the first moment that I formulated something like this without knowing what to call it. I was twenty-two years old when I realized that every single party I went to wound me up much more than was "normal."

What are the advantages and the disadvantages of being highly sensitive?

It's sometimes an advantage being able to pick up on other people's moods. At the same time, that can also be a big disadvantage for me. I can't close my ears, and similarly, I find it very difficult to turn down the degree to which I notice people's moods around me. I find it hard to shut myself off in terms of my mood. It remains a disadvantage that I find it hard to overcome certain things. Going to a party can be a real burden for me, and hosting one is such a big deal for me that I've only hosted three in the last twenty years. The intensity with which one experiences things demands a lot of energy.

Looking back, what sort of messages or feedback would have been helpful to you?

- "It is completely okay to disengage sometimes. You don't have to take part in everything."
- "You can use your high sensitivity."
- "It makes sense to take your high sensitivity into account when you're deciding what career to follow."

What are the particular challenges that highly sensitive men face in our society?

James Bond is not highly sensitive. The masculine image that is propagated in advertisements and films doesn't have anything to do with high sensitivity. Despite the fact that I find all of these things very banal, I can't deny that these things have affected me. I think it is a challenge to accept that you might feel better if you consciously deal with your emotions and the potential limitations in your life. Doing this consciously, but also self-confidently, isn't very easy for me.

How does your high sensitivity impact your relationships with other men?

I feel like it's a limitation that I have difficulties being with people over a long period, whether they're men or women. I find it particularly difficult when there are very few opportunities to take a break. For this reason, I have, for instance, turned down an invitation to my friend's bachelor party. Now that I'm in my early forties, rather than my twenties, this peer pressure hardly plays any kind of role for me, but I used to find it very difficult to deal with my idiosyncrasies. I now find it easier to make sense of this cautiousness. So I don't find it as problematic as I used to, but it is still something that bothers me. Of course, you tend to remain friends with those people who can deal with it or don't give you the feeling that you're a weirdo.

How does high sensitivity impact your relationships with women?

I often had a problem with the fact that I could never fulfill the role of the extroverted, daredevil man that I wanted to be. So the effect that my high sensitivity had on my intimate relationships with women was that I didn't have that many. The "emotional risks" were just too big.

What are the advantages and the disadvantages of being highly sensitive at work?

I didn't consider my high sensitivity at all when I first chose my career. My ambition was too strong, and I wasn't yet able to take my feelings into account. So for a few years, I worked in the commercial sector. This wasn't the right career choice for me for a number of reasons. Aside from the fact that I didn't find the work meaningful, many of the characteristics of high sensitivity were a disadvantage for the work. Making calls and answering emails while the radio was on and my colleagues were chatting—it was just too much.

I now work in an elementary school. I suspect that it's related to my high sensitivity that I can remember really well what it was like for me as a school kid in certain situations. High sensitivity can also be an advantage when it comes to assessing certain moments, issues, and feelings. At the same time, these opportunities can be limited by the fact that I'm often very preoccupied by my own strong feelings.

What's your advice for other highly sensitive men?

I would recommend reading about the phenomenon, taking your own needs seriously, even if they're different to other people's. As a highly sensitive man, exactly how and what one is going to change about one's lifestyle is something that needs to be discovered and tried out over time. We all need to decode our own "user manuals." My advice to other highly sensitive men, and perhaps also to myself, is: whether or not it fits to the propagated image of what a man should be, be confident that you have characteristics that make certain things in life easier and others more difficult.

CHAPTER 9

Self-Worth and Self-Care for Highly Sensitive Men

NOW THAT YOU HAVE READ and learned a lot about emotional regulation, self-soothing, and being attentive to yourself and why these strategies are particularly important for highly sensitive people, I want to take a closer look in this chapter at self-worth and self-care.

Self-worth seems to me to be so important because I've got the impression over the past few years that many—though not all—highly sensitive men suffer from low self-worth and often wish that they had more self-confidence. In my opinion, self-care is closely connected to self-worth because if I believe that I have worth as a person, then it becomes much easier for me to take care of myself and my well-being in my daily life. For instance, in the way that I notice, respect, and verbalize my emotions, my boundaries, and my emotional needs and then take responsibility for myself when I act.

This chapter also builds on the previous chapter and is, I think, a good way to conclude this book because self-care is so closely linked to our behavior as well as to how we interact with others and how we actively and pragmatically shape our lives in this world. While the previous chapter was about internal processes and changes, this chapter is going to be more focused on how you, as a highly sensitive man, can also express these inner changes as external changes in your behavior.

Leading a life that fits our temperament and creating a life and a routine that basically feels good—aside from the normal human highs and lows that we all experience—are also hugely important. At the end of the day, the vast majority of our lives doesn't take place during the few weeks we spend on holiday or those precious forty-eight hours at the weekend, but in the days in between. In between the big plans that we make and the important life events that we look forward to.

But are you, as a highly sensitive man, good at looking after yourself in everyday life? Do you pay enough attention to your physical needs, to your more sensitive nervous system, which perceives and processes environmental stimuli so deeply that you often become quickly emotional, overstimulated, and stressed? Do you get enough relaxation, time out, and quiet in your everyday life so that you're not permanently feeling overstimulated? Do you set clear boundaries in your relationships and in your job, and are you able to say no? These are all questions that relate to good self-care and that we're going to address in the second part of this chapter.

There is, of course, no such thing as having a perfect life (let's not chase after that illusion!), and you're not always going to be great at looking after yourself in every situation. Even when your daily life is going well and you feel like you've achieved a healthy balance between too much and too little stimulation, this feeling doesn't last forever and will need to be renegotiated again and again in the future. At the same time, when it comes to making changes in our everyday lives, we sometimes have more leeway and more opportunities than we realize. But this requires us to treat ourselves with compassion and benevo-

lence. Only then can we develop an attitude that honors how important our emotional and physical welfare is so that we are able to make
it a very important, though not the sole, priority in our lives. Treating
yourself with kindness and taking your highly sensitive welfare seriously in your daily life—and expressing this practically, emotionally,
and intellectually in the way you look after yourself—is the complete
opposite of excessive self-criticism and the refusal to accept the way
that you were born. Excessive self-criticism and not accepting yourself
means that your self-worth is unable to grow and that you will struggle to improve your self-care, creating a vicious circle.

Understanding that the responsibility for your own emotional
and physical welfare as a highly sensitive man lies with you and the
way that you deal with your disposition in everyday life is for many
people a frightening and sometimes even painful step. What you are
giving up is the hope that someone else might one day take responsibility for your welfare or even responsibility for your dissatisfaction
with your life (and who would that even be?). And, perhaps, taking
responsibility for yourself also means giving up the hope that you
will one day be like the other men who aren't highly sensitive.

At the same time, I believe that taking this step toward more self-
responsibility can also be strengthening. It means finally trusting
yourself and expressing clearly to yourself and to others "That
doesn't work for me" or "That's not good for me." This can hugely increase your self-worth and be genuinely liberating. Because, deep
down, only you know what you need in your everyday life and what
you don't, as well as what you are able to change. It is time to trust
your finely tuned self-awareness.

The Challenge of Self-Worth

There are many possible reasons that someone might have low self-
worth, and it can, of course, be a problem for any person, not just
particularly sensitive people. I do, however, get the impression that

self-worth is sometimes particularly problematic for highly sensitive men because in their childhood's they were given the impression that they were not following the rules for being a boy. They were often seen as being too sensitive, too soft, too whiny, or too shy—somehow too different from most other boys or not the way a proper boy should be.

This was true of the client of mine who was struggling with his high sensitivity and who, because of it, had had the sense since he was a child that he "wasn't right" in comparison with other boys. Now an adult, he had recently changed jobs and felt insecure, nervous, and often overstimulated in his new office and wanted to be like the other men in his team—apparently more confident and less sensitive. My client believed that the way he felt in his job proved that he just "didn't have any self-confidence" and that there was some essential part of him missing that all of the men in his team who appeared to be less sensitive seemed to have. Of course, these sort of negative thoughts only served to further undermine his self-worth and fed his internal self-criticism that as a man he was simply "too sensitive." At the same time, he told me that he had never felt particularly confident at any point in his life and actually had no idea what having more self-confidence would even feel like.

Of course, this client wasn't completely wrong. He did lack self-confidence in his new professional setting. He lacked the confidence in his own ability to master the new work situation. We thus started by defining and breaking down what "more self-confident" might mean for him. What it actually meant was:

- Having his inner protector by his side at work and being able to activate him whenever he became aware of his highly sensitive side and noticed that it needed support, acceptance, or encouragement.
- Reminding himself of the positive characteristics and strengths that came from his high sensitivity.
- Recognizing that his expectations were excessively high and trying to reduce them.

- Becoming more active in shaping his relationships with his colleagues and his boss and expressing himself more clearly.
- Leaving on time and taking the necessary time in the evenings to relax.

I mention this example of my client because I think it typifies the way that we so often talk about self-confidence and self-worth in our society—as if one has it or not. As if self-worth were a small, solid object that you were given at some point and stuck in your pocket, and it could be pulled out every time that things looked a bit dicey.

If you watch reality shows on TV now and again, you'll often see the jury saying to the stressed and nervous candidates, "You just have to have more self-confidence!" It sounds so easy, as if they just have to remember that that hard little object is in their pocket and they just have to reach in and pull it out. As if those poor contestants just had to "pull themselves together." In reality, it seems to me that the ability to have confidence in oneself and to judge oneself positively and as being of worth is much more complicated and complex—a soft, fluid object that quickly changes shape, sometimes grows, sometimes shrinks, is sometimes easy to get hold of, and is sometimes much harder to grasp.

It is, of course, desirable to feel self-confident (and, lest we forget, as a man very much desired by society—that traditional masculine ideal again) and to be aware of our worth as a person because it's good for our psychological health and, in general, makes life much easier. And yet I'm really not sure that it is the panacea that it is often made out to be. Because we now know that while having too little self-worth isn't good for people, having too much can also be problematic for people because it doesn't protect us from engaging in problematic behavior and it can often be accompanied by narcissism, aggression, violent behavior, self-aggrandizement, and interpersonal conflict.[1,2,3] I suspect that we have all met a few examples of this kind of person.

Perhaps it's less about having *a lot* of self-worth and more about having *enough*. This would mean judging yourself and your own sensitivity positively and being aware enough of your own worth that you are able to shape your own life and relationships to fit your desires, values, preferences, and emotional needs. To feel worthwhile enough as a man that you can generally live well with it. Free, self-sufficient, and calm.

I'm raising these things because I believe that the public discourse around self-worth and self-confidence is far too simplistic. In my work as a therapist, I often notice that this leads to many people—particularly those who are less self-confident—chasing after the pretty empty, unrealistic, and dishonest idea of self-confidence that is sometimes propagated by the media.

It is important here to pay attention to your own inner monologue. If you hear often enough from other people that you don't have enough self-confidence, then at some point this will become a set part of your personal narrative and one that you begin to tell yourself. Are you then even going to be able to notice when you do feel a sense of self-worth or when you have acted in a self-confident way in a particular situation?

It is, of course, vital that you address self-worth if you believe that you might be a highly sensitive man who has problems with your self-worth because of your sensitivity and the effects it had on you when you were growing up, and if you believe that this clearly had a detrimental impact on your life, causes you pain, and limits you. You need to see your sensitive aptitudes in a more positive light, creating a relationship with yourself that is less critical, less demanding, and less perfectionistic.

But I also think that it is worth us thinking about what the term *self-worth* actually means for you. If you equate "becoming more self-confident" with "being less sensitive," then I think you're likely to fall into a trap that's going to be hard to get out of. What is also important to realize is that self-worth and also the sources of our self-worth can change over the course of our lives. Our self-worth can relate to certain areas of our lives and not to others; it can be something we're sometimes more and sometimes less conscious of;

it is dependent on context, time, people, and whomever we're comparing ourselves to.[4] Self-worth is dynamic, it's alive, and it's not
necessarily something that's fixed.

Try to think about in which areas of your life, with which people,
and at which times you *already* feel confident and have worth, as well
as in which areas this is not the case. Might it be possible that, in certain areas, you have always been much more self-confident than you
think and than your inner monologue has given you credit for over
the years? Do you perhaps do things that come completely naturally
to you, but that other people wouldn't have the confidence to do?

Every step toward having more self-worth goes hand in hand with
being attentive to yourself in an accepting, mindful, and compassionate way and with the solid and practical self-care that goes along with
it. These two things represent the foundations of self-worth.

Self-Worth as a Highly Sensitive Man and Working with the Inner Critic

In everyday speech, terms such as *self-worth, feelings of self-worth, self-
confidence*, and *self-assurance* are often used interchangeably. It can
thus often seem difficult to clearly separate and define these terms.
All of these concepts are at heart about how people judge and esti-
mate themselves and their own abilities and accomplishments and
how they see these things in relation to other people. The psychologists Friederike Potreck-Rose and Gitta Jacob offer the following
explanation: "Self-confidence is particularly related to the conviction that one can do something. Self-worth goes beyond this and
includes, for instance, the estimation of personal attributes that are
not necessarily related to competence. As such, self-confidence can
be understood as being a component of self-worth, which is focused
on competence and proficiency."[5]

Both Potreck-Rose and Jacob believe that a solid sense of self-
worth is held up by four columns:

1. **SELF-ACCEPTANCE:** Having a positive, benevolent, and accepting attitude to yourself, meaning accepting yourself as a competent person just as you are, with your own personal weaknesses and defects.
2. **SELF-CONFIDENCE:** Believing in your own achievements and skills and assessing these positively; for instance, knowing what you're good at and what you're not good at.
3. **SOCIAL COMPETENCE:** Being able to make secure social contacts and develop them in a way that is acceptable to you. This means being able to negotiate intimacy and distance to other people, to maintain a good interpersonal exchange, to read social signals, and to recognize what is required of social situations.
4. **SOCIAL NETWORK:** Feeling socially integrated and, because of this, feeling that your own fundamental emotional need for intimacy is being satisfied. This means being part of a group, maintaining friendships and romantic relationships, and feeling secure and safe with other people.

I wanted to outline these components of self-worth because I think they show very clearly that having a solid sense of self-worth is, in part, based on our attitude about ourselves and our abilities and achievements, but is also partly based on factors outside of ourselves, namely in the interpersonal: our contacts and experiences with and connections to other people.

The majority of highly sensitive men that I have met are completely socially competent and often have a good (if at times small) social network. The reason for this, I believe, lies with the particular qualities of highly sensitive men: their very precise interpersonal awareness, their need for depth, their high capacity for empathy, how observant they are to subtle social signals and messages, and the deep emotional and intellectual processing that takes place in their interaction with the other person. All of these are positive characteristics that highly sensitive men have and that others appreciate in them. I'm certain of that. Who among us wouldn't want to feel that the person we're talking to is fully engaged emotionally and intellectually and in a compassionate way with what we're saying? To be seen and heard by the person we're engaging with?

Self-acceptance and self-confidence are, however, generally much more problematic for many highly sensitive men. As mentioned above, I believe that this is related to the fact that many highly sensitive men already felt as boys that they did not fit the norm. Their self-acceptance and self-confidence have thus often been undermined by the explicit and implicit feedback they received from their social surroundings. These highly sensitive men often develop a particularly critical part of themselves, which I would like to call their "inner critic." This is, of course, a simplification of a very complex psychological process.

Maybe a few of you will recognize this inner critic who, throughout the day, criticizes your behavior, your appearance, your sensitive nature, sometimes your whole person, or makes excessive demands of you. He will often say things like "The way you are is not okay," "You're an embarrassment, everyone can see it," "You're so unfit," "You're too sensitive," "You're weak," "Your body should be slimmer/more muscular/more attractive," "Everyone else is self-confident except for you," "Weakling," "You're not a real man," "You've not been successful enough in your career," and so on and so on.

If you, as a highly sensitive man, want to increase your self-acceptance and self-confidence, then you have to try to shut off this inner critic more often and use your inner protector to recognize and challenge these excessively self-critical thoughts. Is what my inner critic telling me really true? What would my inner protector say in this situation? The more mindfully you deal with yourself, the quicker you will notice when the critical part of you is making himself heard and the quicker you will be able to react and fight back.

Assuming that the tone and content of your inner critic isn't too destructive, cruel or punishing, for many of you the goal here may actually be to isolate him more quickly or not to let him speak as often instead of completely getting rid of him. It may be the case that your inner critic isn't always just trying to be cruel and is sometimes hoping that his critical comments are protecting you from greater harm: "You need to knuckle down at work (then your boss won't criticize you as much and your colleagues will like you more)." "Maybe it's best to keep quiet (so that no one will laugh at you)." "Don't be so sure of yourself (pride goeth before a fall)." What can really help here is recognizing the desire that sits behind the criticism and, with the help of your inner protector, reformulating it.

1. What is your inner critic trying to do? What is his aim?
2. Do I also want what the inner critic wants? If not, what do I want instead?
3. Will what my inner critic is saying bring me closer to this goal?
4. If not, what could I say to myself instead? How could I express it differently?
5. How would my inner protector formulate that?

But if your inner critic is very disparaging and rejects your sensitive side as a highly sensitive man, or is embarrassed by it, even, then you need to take action because he can really inhibit your sense of self-worth. This is why you need your inner protector—the loving father, the supportive friend, the consolatory side of yourself, whatever you want to call it—who, as a foil to your inner critic, is always by your side. Because his goal is to treat you well and to bolster your self-confidence and your self-acceptance. Unlike your inner critic, he likes your sensitivity and he likes you exactly the way you are.

Let's practice creating a dialogue between your critical side and your protective, accepting side. This exercise also works well as a journal that you can keep over many days and weeks. Every time during the day that your inner critic gets in touch, jot down a couple of sentences recording exactly what he said. Then think about what

Dialogue Between Your Inner Critic and Your Inner Protector

TIME AND DATE	ACTIVITY/ SITUATION	INNER CRITIC'S COMMENT	INNER PROTECTOR'S ANSWER
Monday, 10:00 am	A colleague was talking about his weekend and mentioned his big group of friends.	"Unlike you, this guy's popular and active. You just sat around at home again and wasted your precious time. No wonder no one likes you."	"What a load of baloney. That's not true at all. You had a difficult week, and you needed some peace and quiet. This is important for you, and I think it's great that you took some time out. You are fine just the way you are, and your friends like you."

your inner protector would say to this. Pay particular attention to the moment in which your inner critic demeans or criticizes your sensitivity. A number of my clients who have practiced this exercise regularly over a long period tell me that, after a while, their inner protector begins to develop a range of standard responses, such as "No, that's not right" or "Stop, I don't want to hear that anymore."

Resources and Strengths

To strengthen your sense of self-confidence, it is a good idea to become more conscious of your own abilities, to see them more positively, and to have more faith in them. So in the next exercise, I want to take a closer look at your individual resources and strengths. By that, I mean those areas, achievements, and abilities that you connect with contentment, pleasure, and well-being and that make you stand out and make you who you are. (If your inner critic pipes up at any point during this exercise, then let him know that he's banned from speaking for the rest of the chapter.)

Give yourself some time to complete this exercise and try to answer in as much detail as possible. You can also complete it over a number of days and keep coming back to it to add to it. Then try the following: take another a look at what you wrote above, and using the prompts below, write down which of the strengths, experiences, and qualities that you noted above are related to your highly sensitive temperament.

Qualities and Strengths

What do you like about yourself (abilities, characteristics, beliefs, appearance, qualities, etc.)?	
What can you do well (talents, abilities, professionally, interpersonally, etc.)?	
What makes you feel content and gives you a sense of inner calm in your life (places, activities, people, hobbies, animals, nature, etc.)?	
With which areas of your life are you pretty content or even very content at the moment (job, friendships, relationships, appearance, free time, etc.)?	

When, during which activities, and with which people do you feel self-confident, secure, and authentic?	
Which events, achievements, or relationships in your life are you particularly proud of?	
What difficulties and challenges in your life have you overcome? Which characteristics, talents, and qualities in your life helped you to overcome these challenges?	
What do other people particularly like about you? (Ask three people whom you trust to name three positive characteristics about you.)	
If your teenage self could see you today, what would he like about you and your life? What would he be happy about? What would he be amazed by?	

1. Which of the above-mentioned strengths and qualities are directly or partly a consequence of my high sensitivity?

   _____

   _____

   _____

2. What are the positive consequences of my high sensitivity that I'm particularly thankful for?

   _____

   _____

   _____

3. When and how do I use the positive characteristics of my high sensitivity in my everyday life, in my relationships, and in my career?

   _____

   _____

   _____

4. When and in which situations do I feel most comfortable with my highly sensitive temperament?

_____

_____

_____

5. Which people in my life give me the feeling that they accept and value me as a highly sensitive man?

_____

_____

_____

6. When and in which ways could I use and enjoy my highly sensitive characteristics in my everyday life more often?

_____

_____

_____

7. Sketch out a future version of your life in which you live contentedly and authentically, in tune with your sensitive temperament. Pay particular attention to areas such as work, everyday life, relationships, friendships, and free time. What would your life look like?

_____

_____

_____

Strategies to Improve Self-Care

As I explained at the beginning of the chapter, when we talk about self-care, we mean the ability to look after and look out for ourselves in our everyday lives as highly sensitive men. This means dealing well with things intellectually, emotionally, and behaviorally. This is not always going to work perfectly, but when we treat ourselves with an inner attitude of acceptance, warmth, compassion, kindness, and care, and feel our worth as highly sensitive men, then these are the best foundations for good self-care.

Despite all of our differences and our diversity, there are also many similarities in terms of what is good for highly sensitive men and what isn't. This means that however differently you lead your life, however different the experiences of your sensitivity have been—which will, in turn, have influenced your life, your personality, and your attitudes—the four DOES indicators (depth of processing; over-stimulation; emotional reactivity, including empathy; sensitivity to subtle stimuli) can still guide you in what you need to be aware of in everyday life and how to orient your self-care.

I have met many highly sensitive men over the past few years who live a life that would be a good fit for someone who was not highly sensitive, but that for them leads to recurrent problems, such as irritability, heightened anxiety, problems sleeping, chronic over-stimulation, and symptoms of depression. The reason for this, as I see it, is nearly always an attitude to self-care that completely ignores these four DOES indicators.

I therefore want us to look at different areas of life and to give you some concrete self-care strategies for each of these areas, all of which would be important for anyone, but are particularly so for highly sensitive people. I'm not trying to help you avoid situations in your life that you don't like or that you find challenging. Of course, one sometimes needs to face difficult situations and challenging feelings in order to learn how to better deal with them in the future and to achieve positive, long-term goals. What I want to do here, instead, is to support you in giving yourself permission to live your life and to care for yourself in a way that genuinely does you good. To allow you to live your life authentically and well as a highly sensitive man. I have put together the following (in no way exhaustive) list of recommendations with my clients over the years, which I'm sure many of you will be able to use in your own lives. Try to see this list as food for thought in terms of how you might be able to better deal with your high sensitivity in your daily life. Use my suggestions as inspiration for your own ideas and be creative.

Strategies and Ideas for Good Self-Care for Highly Sensitive People

1. EVERYDAY LIFE AND ORGANIZING YOUR FREE TIME

- **MAKE RELAXATION AND RECOVERY A PRIORITY IN YOUR LIFE.** You now know that you feel overstimulated more quickly and more often and thus become more overaroused than most other people. This means that you need more time out and regular opportunities for relaxation. Try to use at least one day in the week for complete relaxation. No duties, no parties, no shopping, no crowds, no overstimulation. On this day, only do things that you find physically, spiritually, and emotionally relaxing and calming, whether that means staying in bed, reading, going for a walk, painting, listening to music, relaxing, working in the garden, playing a sport, seeking out quiet or contemplative places (a church, a museum, a gallery, etc.) or going swimming. Whatever it is, allow yourself this conscious period of relaxation. You're not being lazy or unproductive; you're simply paying attention to your particularly sensitive nervous system and your physical needs.
- **SLEEP.** Your body recovers best during sleep. Therefore make sure, particularly during the week, that you're getting enough sleep and that you're maintaining a healthy sleep routine (not drinking alcohol or coffee before going to bed, going to bed at the same time every night, having a cool and dark bedroom, maintaining a relaxing and calming evening routine before you go to bed, perhaps wearing earplugs or a sleep mask, etc.). Work out what your individ-

ual sleep needs are—usually around eight hours—and try to stick with them as much as possible.

- **TRANSPORTATION.** If you have to regularly take public transportation, then think about whether there's a quieter alternative route that you could take or whether, for instance, there's an earlier or later connection that you might find more pleasant. Perhaps you could walk or ride a bike. You might also want to use earplugs or headphones if you have problems with sensitivity to subtle stimuli on public transportation. Use the "Quiet Zone" in the train. If you have to travel by car, then try to create a calm atmosphere by, for instance, turning off the radio the moment you feel stressed, making sure the car smells good, and keeping it at the right temperature. If you are flying, then think about which seat you generally find most pleasant (back or front, aisle or window).
- **SHOPPING AND GOING OUT.** Seek out restaurants, cafes, bars, and shops that have a quiet and relaxed atmosphere, perhaps because they're particularly cozy, are well lit, or are usually emptier, less hectic, or quieter. When you're reserving a table in a busy restaurant, specifically ask for a table in a quiet corner, particularly on those days that you're already feeling overstimulated. Strategically use quiet times of the day. Go to the movies in the afternoon or go shopping in the evening. I often get the sense that online shopping is a complete godsend for a huge number of highly sensitive people.
- **EATING AND DRINKING.** Eat three regular meals a day and have small snacks in between so that you don't get low blood sugar—something that you likely are sensitive to. Drink enough liquids throughout the day. Pay attention to how much caffeine and alcohol you can take and whether you should avoid either.
- **TIME ALONE.** Make sure you're spending time alone regularly and that you're doing it in a space that isn't

overstimulating, unless you find it unpleasant to be alone. You could find this time during your journey to work or perhaps by taking walks. You might consider taking a few minutes out in the morning before work or in the evening when you come home, before you start cooking or chatting to your loved ones.

- **NATURE.** Most highly sensitive people find contact with nature particularly calming and relaxing. Try to use this resource whenever it's available to you. Take walks, spend time in the garden, read a book in the park, or take a drive to the nearest wood, lake, river, or beach.
- **VACATIONS.** Take regular vacations and organize them in such a way that they are actually relaxing for you. Make sure you don't let too much time elapse between vacations. If possible, you might want to try to take some time off every three months or so in a quiet environment close to nature.
- **HOME.** Make your home a place of calm in which you feel completely comfortable, secure, relaxed, and safe. Make it as beautiful as you can; you, as a highly sensitive person, will particularly profit from creating a quiet and pleasant environment that fits your temperament. If this isn't possible, then you should at least create a room or at the very least a quiet corner of a room that you can retreat to; for instance, on a comfy armchair with a soft blanket where you can get cozy.
- **SHORT BREAKS.** Over the course of your day, try to take regular small breaks between work and other duties. Notice your breathing, close your eyes, and relax your body without trying to do something else at the same time. Try to turn off your telephone for short periods and every now and again try to give yourself "electronics breaks." Find a quiet space when you notice that you feel tense, stressed, and overstimulated, and you long for less stimulation. When you need a short break, you could dip into a church,

walk along a quiet street, sit in a small park, or find a quiet corner in a bookshop or library. It might even be as simple as stopping on your way to the bathroom or closing the door to your office.

- **SENSITIVITY TO SUBTLE STIMULI.** Pay attention to your sensory sensitivity and get creative. Cut the labels out of your clothes if you don't like the way they feel on your skin. Only buy clothes made of fabrics that you like the feel of. Use earplugs and sleep masks whenever you need to. Change your light bulbs at home to ones with warmer and softer light. Use candles, natural light, or multiple small sources of light in your home, rather than one very bright overhead lamp. Turn off the radio, TV, or computer when you notice that it all feels like too much. But also use the advantages of your sensitivity to subtle stimuli. Listen to music to positively influence your mood. Regularly treat yourself to massages. Go swimming or notice how your body feels when you're engaged in sports. Find an essential oil that you find particularly calming and pleasant and keep it with you. On your desk or on your cell phone screen, keep photos of people or places that are important to you. Hang up pictures around your home that really speak to you or move you. Enjoy your sex life and the physical intensity connected with it. Spend time in places that you particularly respond to and that you find particularly beautiful. Really use all of your five senses very consciously whenever you can.

- **MINDFULNESS AND RELAXATION.** Regularly practice mindfulness, physical relaxation, and imagery exercises. Make activities like meditation, yoga, and sports a regular part of your daily routine.

- **STRUCTURE AND ROUTINE.** How much structure do you need in everyday life to feel good? Routine and repetition can sometimes be calming because they create predictability.

Of course, too much structure can quickly lead to rigidity and, in turn, to a loss of vitality in your life.

- **ACCEPTANCE.** However many breaks and however much calm you build into your everyday life, you are always going to be faced with overstimulation. These are the moments to practice acceptance, to relax your body, and to listen to your inner protector. ("This will be over soon. You can tolerate this. Relax—we're going to get through this.")

- **ENJOY YOURSELF AND SEEK OUT POSITIVE STIMULI AND EXPERIENCES.** Enjoy your highly sensitive temperament and your rich inner life. Enjoy that you process stimuli more deeply. Be happy that positive things can quickly relax you, give you pleasure, and make you think, whether it's reading books, watching films, taking part in discussions, chatting with friends, or reflecting on a real situation. Notice all of the pleasant details in your daily life, which you notice quicker and more consciously than less sensitive people— delicious food, a smile, a sunset, the wind on your skin, the smell of the streets after rain, the rustle of leaves, luminous colors, a lovely moment with another person, the glitter of the snow, the singing of birds, bright flowers in a vase. Consciously seek out positive stimuli that you can concentrate on. What is beautiful in this moment? What do I notice that I find pleasant and positive?

- **IMPROVING THE SITUATION.** In difficult moments, ask yourself what you could change to make the situation more pleasant or easier to bear. What do you need physically or emotionally to feel better? What would good self-care look like in this moment? How could you talk to yourself and support yourself in this situation? I'm thinking here about very practical changes (breathing deeply and consciously relaxing your body, opening a window, turning down the radio, drinking a glass of water), but also about more subtle internal changes (self-compassion, self-acceptance, consciously dealing with yourself in a kind way, or giving yourself the courage to accept the situation instead of rejecting it).

- **SPEAKING TO OTHER PEOPLE ABOUT YOUR SENSITIVE NATURE.** Only you and you alone can decide whom you tell about your particularly sensitive nature and whom you don't tell. When you do decide to share, pay attention to the context, to whether you trust the person, and to how much you want to disclose. If, for whatever reason, you don't want to use the term high sensitivity when speaking to other people about it, you can instead say, for instance, "That doesn't fit my temperament." Or stick to expressing your (highly sensitive) needs without using the words highly sensitive. You can say, for instance, "I prefer it when it's not so full," "I need lots of time alone," or "Let's go somewhere else. I find it a bit too loud in here."

2. WORK

- **WORKING HOURS.** Arrive and leave punctually and avoid overtime. I know that overtime is either demanded or at least celebrated in many workplaces, and perhaps your inner critic likes you to have a high workload as a measure of your self-worth. But I think that the price you pay for this is just too high. I know highly sensitive men who have strategically reduced their working hours (and accepted earning less money in return) or who have found a new job that offers them more control and flexibility when it comes to their working hours. If you don't feel able or don't want to do this, then at least aim to leave the office on time. Work is an important part of life, but at the end of the day it is just one part.
- **LUNCH BREAK.** Make sure that you regularly take and fully exploit your lunch break. Leave your desk and spend your break somewhere that allows you a little distance and

room to relax. You might want to take a walk around the block, find a quiet café, or even create a quiet corner at your workplace by, for instance, closing the door to your office, dimming the lights, putting your phone on silent, or lying on the floor of your office for a few minutes (if, of course, you have your own office). Be creative. I had one highly sensitive client who always spent his lunch break in the nearest park—come rain or shine. If you usually have lunch in a noisy cafeteria or restaurant with your colleagues and you find it stressful, then allow yourself not to join in or at least to sit it out now and again.

- **STRUCTURE AND MULTITASKING.** As much as you can, try to avoid multitasking and try instead to complete one task after the other. At the beginning or end of the day, write yourself a to-do list. Order tasks by how important and urgent they are. Try to be realistic about what you can get done and reward yourself with something small when you have completed your tasks. It's better to keep this list short and achievable instead of coming home frustrated every day because you haven't been able to work through an unrealistic list.

- **CAREER CHOICE.** Our careers can't be a calling for every one of us. For many of us, our job is primarily about earning enough money to live on. And there are many ways to find meaning and fulfillment in our lives outside of work. So when you are choosing which career path to follow, think carefully about the positive characteristics, skills, and qualities that go hand in hand with your temperamental traits. My friend Oliver (see chapter 3) is a good example of how important our professional setting and environment is for our highly sensitive welfare. It is likely that you will find common work stresses particularly difficult to bear, such as tight deadlines, team conflicts, a difficult boss, loud open-plan offices, long team meetings, and chaotic and constantly changing working conditions that are impossible to plan for. Where possible, try to use all the opportunities and freedoms that you have at your work in your favor. For Oliver, this means working freelance; for others, it might mean relocating, finding a quieter desk, talking openly with colleagues to deal with a conflict, or even avoiding large team meetings where possible. There is, of course, no such thing as the perfect workplace, but that doesn't mean that your working conditions and environment have to be in complete opposition to your sensitivity. I have met many highly sensitive men who spent far too long in a job or professional environment that didn't suit their temperament, and they paid a high price for it with their frustration, self-doubt, exhaustion, symptoms of depression, and increased anxiety.

- **INNER PROTECTOR, MINDFULNESS, AND RELAXATION.** Always remember that your compassionate and calming self is always with you and that you can always turn to your inner protector for advice and support. Maybe your inner protector has to remind you more often of the strengths and positive characteristics that go hand in hand with your high sensitivity. Practice mindfulness and conscious physical relaxation—particularly in challenging and stressful work situations.

3. RELATIONSHIPS, FRIENDSHIPS, AND SOCIAL CONTACTS

- **BE AUTHENTIC.** You are who you are, and you are allowed to be who you are. Don't try to be something you're not. This might sound banal, but it's actually much harder to do than you might think. Whether it's your partner, friends, relatives, or parents, don't let anyone tell you that as a man you aren't allowed to be sensitive, thoughtful, deep, and emotional and that you don't need time out and help from others. This message is simply wrong, and, what's more, it's unhealthy. I believe that authenticity is something that makes people particularly attractive and that we feel most comfortable in our own skin when we have authentic contact with other people. I get the impression that particularly sensitive people are often naturally very authentic. Use and look after this strength.

- **FIND YOUR OWN WAY TO CHALLENGE TRADITIONAL MASCULINE STEREOTYPES.** If dealing authentically and creatively with your high sensitivity doesn't fit the image of a typical man, then this is a great opportunity to challenge and expand this antiquated image, with all of its unhealthy and narrow rules and norms about what being a man means. I believe that reminding yourself of this again and again can be really helpful.

- **IN YOUR RELATIONSHIPS AND FRIENDSHIPS, SAY NO MORE OFTEN AND MAKE SURE YOU HAVE ENOUGH FREEDOM.** Other people, and our relationships with them, can sometimes be intense, tiring, and overstimulating, particularly when you are both highly sensitive and introverted. If you have a tendency to subordinate yourself or to look for excessive recognition from people, then this can become really problematic. Allow yourself to say no more often and, in doing so, to verbalize your boundaries to other people. It is one thing to notice when our boundaries are being crossed; it is another to express this to other people and, in doing so, to give yourself more respect. So the next time you're invited out, are offered a job, or are asked for help, just say no if you really feel that it's going to overstimulate you or that it's not going to fit your temperament. In your relationships, express clearly, but also sensitively, how you feel and what you need emotionally from the other person or from the situation. This might mean, for example, saying more clearly that you need time alone or more space.

- **USE YOUR SENSITIVITY TO CREATE CLOSE AND SECURE CONNECTIONS.** Use the positive interpersonal characteristics and qualities—such as sensitivity and empathy—that go hand in hand with your high sensitivity to build and maintain trusting and close connections with others. Trust your highly sensitive "tool" when it comes to interpersonal contact. Seek out confidantes and allies in your life—whether or not they're highly sensitive—who like you and value you and in whose presence you feel respected, secure, and liked as a highly sensitive man.

- **MAKE CONTACT WITH OTHER HIGHLY SENSITIVE PEOPLE.** I think that contact with other highly sensitive people can be really important, and you can take part in a workshop, a retreat, or a self-help group, or use the internet to get in touch with other men like you. You will likely discover many similarities, but also many differences. Even if the differences overweigh the similarities, you will still get the sense that you are not alone with your temperamental trait and that there are others who self-identify as particularly sensitive in temperament as well. Making an effort to get in touch with other highly sensitive men can also be really important so that you can talk openly about your experiences as a highly sensitive man.

- **BE A HIGHLY SENSITIVE ROLE MODEL.** This may be easier if you have your own children, but even if you don't have any kids, you can still be a great role model for sensitive and emotional masculinity. You can show your nieces, nephews, godchildren, and the children of friends and acquaintances that being a man is multifaceted and multilayered and that men are also allowed to be sensitive, compassionate, deep, cautious, introverted, and emotional. Also be a role model for other men by signaling that for you feelings and deep thoughts are not only welcome, but actually wanted.

Summary

It is, of course, difficult to offer blanket tips and strategies for good self-care when, despite all of their similarities, highly sensitive men are a heterogeneous group with different lives, relationships, values, and experiences. What for one of you might be a good way of living and a kind of self-care that works, might not necessarily work for someone else. At the end of the day, only you know what you need in a given situation and in which situations you need to pay more attention to yourself.

I believe, though, that you can trust yourself in this process precisely because you feel so much, you think about things so deeply, and your perception is so discriminating and sensitive. Always think about the fact that this doesn't just bring disadvantages. Quite the opposite. Because, unlike less sensitive people, you notice very quickly when something isn't working for you or when something does or doesn't feel right. But more than this, I also believe that it comes very naturally to you to think a lot about how you might solve these apparent problems. As a highly sensitive man, you can really trust this characteristic of yours.

And so we return to the issue of self-confidence: trusting enough that deep down you know and can sense what is good for you and which concrete changes you need to make in your daily life. And also that you have enough self-confidence in your own skills and capabilities to convert this perception into practical changes and behaviors.

Sebastian: "Crying, laughing, and the expression of every other emotion is as normal for a man as it is for a woman."

Sebastian is forty years old, works as a music producer, and is a father to three sons. He is a really clear example of how having knowledge about your own high sensitivity can help you to recognize the patterns in your own life.

When and how did you first notice you were highly sensitive?

I first understood that I was highly sensitive around the age of forty. I read Elaine Aron's book, and all the pieces fell into place. My childhood and my entire life up to the age of forty suddenly all made sense, and I could, for the first time in my life, have a clear and profound understanding of my behavior up until that point. This was an immense relief. A lot of the restlessness I've had throughout my entire life settled, and I could finally see and distinguish behavioral and emotional patterns I have, choices I have made. All this led to a sense of ease and actually forgiving myself. It was like a big sigh of relief.

What are the advantages and the disadvantages of being highly sensitive?

One disadvantage of being highly sensitive for me is that I never really bonded or identified with other men because I felt so different from them. Therefore, I seek and have a lot more fulfilling friendships with women. I never felt comfortable in groups and always preferred having one real friend as opposed to having many acquaintances. Another disadvantage is getting easily overstimulated in public or in loud places, like clubs, trains, subways, or other small, confined places with a lot of people in them. I can rarely stand being in such places for very long. And finally, having strong emotions can feel overwhelming, and I sometimes feel "drenched" by my own feelings.

But there are also many advantages to being highly sensitive. For instance, being very creative, having a strong inner life, and an abundance of ideas. Everything tastes and feels more pronounced, and I am basically constantly in a state of awe. I have great attention to detail and notice even tiny changes in my surroundings. My perception of others is very nuanced, as I notice changes in their moods, feelings, tone of voice, or the emotional quality of what they are saying very quickly. I feel people almost like a sponge, but that can be a double-edged sword sometimes.

How does high sensitivity impact on your relationships with other men?

I find the company of other men, especially in groups, very difficult, sometimes. I get the impression that, in order to be masculine, you need to be loud, insensitive, and must enjoy doing "manly" things. I rarely do small talk as I get bored immediately, and if I cannot change the topic of conversation to something more personal or emotional, I usually leave the situation, if that's possible. I think nowadays other men appreciate my high sensitivity, but I think that has a lot to do with me accepting myself as being highly sensitive. Nevertheless, I am very particular with whom I choose to share that information. I do not tell everyone that I'm highly sensitive.

How does high sensitivity impact on your relationships with women?

When it comes to forming friendships or relationships with women, I find being highly sensitive a huge advantage. I get the sense that women are usually much more emotionally developed and emotionally intelligent than men, which makes me a lot more inclined to talk to them. I have been attracting women easily throughout my life, and I think my sensitivity has been a big reason for this. When it comes to sexual encounters, I need to have an emotional connection with the woman before sleeping with her, otherwise it feels pointless to me.

What are the challenges of being a highly sensitive father?

I am very attuned to the emotional states of my children, even if I don't always express it. One thing that is very important to me is to never scold them in public. It's always counterproductive, always. I can feel when they are not happy or have done something that they shouldn't have, and I try to find ways to communicate with them that are nonconfrontational, as this relieves them from feeling shame and guilt. This means that I can easily motivate them to open up and to share with me what's going on. Communicating with them in a sensitive way, so that they don't feel judged or accused, also helps when we all need to cooperate on a task. They are more inclined to want to help, rather than feel they "have to."

What are the advantages and the disadvantages of being highly sensitive at work?

At work, colleagues tend to engage in small talk, whereas I like to have meaningful conversations with them. When this happens, I usually move to different parts of my workplace where I can spend time on my own. I enjoy my exchanges with customers as they usually quickly open up and feel relaxed in my presence and share personal details. When I work as a music producer, I am quickly aware of what makes the artist nervous or anxious. This helps me create a relaxed and comfortable atmosphere in the studio, and the recording session becomes playful and not too formal. I also think that my high sensitivity helps me when it comes to the creative process of making music. I hear instantly when a song is too long or too short, when elements of the musical arrangements are too quiet, loud, or repetitive. I am very aware of all those fine details.

Being highly sensitive, what do you struggle with the most in daily life?

What I struggle with most in everyday life is sensitivity to subtle stimuli and overstimulation. That is my biggest challenge, especially when I work at the store, which is noisy, full of people, with bright lights, music playing, and big windows, with people and cars going by, colleagues or customers asking questions, often at the same time. I feel bombarded with all the stimulation. When I feel overwhelmed, I usually do a breathing exercise or try to center myself by finding a quiet space in the store. Sometimes I lock myself in the toilet for a few minutes and take some deep breaths. I also prefer to eat lunch on my own, often wearing headphones, listening to ambient music or white noise, which relaxes me.

What are your self-care strategies, and what lifestyle changes have you made?

I enjoy sensory touch, and although I often find this intense, it is also relaxing. Therefore, I've started booking monthly massages, which give me an important moment of calm. Having a routine also puts me at ease. I go for a run twice a week in a forest near my house, where I am completely on my own and feel very little stimulation. I find listening to the sounds of the forest very soothing, and regular exercise helps me to de-stress.

Looking back, what sort of messages or feedback would have been helpful to you?

"I love you and I'm proud of you, exactly the way you are." "There's nothing missing or lacking." "Crying, laughing, and the expression of every other emotion is as normal for a man as it is for a woman."

What's your advice for other highly sensitive men?

Embrace your sensitivity and become comfortable with it. Find other highly sensitive people and talk about your feelings and your experiences of being highly sensitive. If you want to function in your everyday life in an intelligent and satisfying way, make downtime an absolute priority and schedule it in several times a week. Share with the people closest to you how you function and what you need, so that you create an environment and social circle that can understand and support you. Personally, sharing with my workplace that I'm highly sensitive made an enormous difference because being open with it helped me to feel less stressed at work.

CHAPTER 10

Conclusions

W E HAVE ARRIVED AT THE end of this book. In my introduction, I expressed the wish that you would feel empowered by this book to try to accept yourself exactly the way you are and that you would learn how you can look after yourself as a highly sensitive man in your everyday life. I hope I've managed to do both things.

It was important for me to illuminate high sensitivity at both the macro and the micro levels. What I mean by that is to look, on the one hand, at the bigger picture in terms of how the term is classified theoretically, psychologically, and scientifically, and how you as a sensitive man are helping change the traditional, sometimes problematic image of the "strong man" in society. The next generation of young men who are growing up now urgently need more freedom and more diversity in terms of what it means to be a man, and they will undoubtedly thank you. On the other hand, it was also important to me to look, on the small scale, at how high sensitivity feels and how it manifests itself completely individually and how you can get better at dealing with your own sensitive disposition in a practical way.

Don't reduce yourself exclusively to a single temperamental trait. There are many temperamental traits and countless influences on our lives that shape and change us. Sometimes the temptation to reduce ourselves to our highly sensitive temperaments is so strong because it can give us an identity and can make us feel special in a world that often seems to demand that we put ourselves into clear categories. Perhaps we hope or rather wish that a single truth can explain our lives—all of our problems, all of our difficulties, all of our foibles. It's just too tempting. And yet it seems important to me that you do recognize your own high sensitivity, that you understand it and accept it so that you can live well with it and thrive.

You must also never forget that you are not alone with the challenges and assets that high sensitivity offers. There are many other men and women who are similar to you. You are in good company. At the end of the day, high sensitivity is an invitation—an invitation to live your own precious and fleeting life with genuine depth and intensity. To intensely deal intellectually and emotionally with yourself, with other people, and the world, and through this to react strongly to positive experiences, situations, and relationships. To allow yourself to be genuinely moved by the world and by life. What a gift! So enjoy and use your high sensitivity to the fullest whenever you can, and at the same time look after yourself. Go out into the world, find your own voice, and seek out allies with whom you can be your authentic self and who like, support, and value your sensitive and emotional masculinity. Because worth, as we have seen, is something that the highly sensitive man undeniably has.

A Conversation with Elaine Aron About Highly Sensitive Men

ELAINE ARON, PH.D., is a clinical psychologist and the leading international academic on high sensitivity. She has decisively shaped the field of sensitivity since 1991 with her research into sensory processing sensitivity, triggering a wave of research into the field. Alongside her academic and therapeutic work, she is also the bestselling author of numerous books on high sensitivity and was involved in the production of the documentary *Sensitive* in 2015. Her first book, *The Highly Sensitive Person*, was published in 1996 and has gone on to sell over a million copies. It has been translated into seventy different languages and is the standard work on high sensitivity.[1]

It became clear over the course of our conversation that the subject of highly sensitive men is a topic that is close to Elaine Aron's heart. She was more than ready to share her expert knowledge and observations about highly sensitive men with me and also to reveal how she personally deals with the overarousal that goes hand in hand with too much stimulation.

TOM FALKENSTEIN: Elaine, thank you so much for talking to me today about highly sensitive men. Before we talk about highly sensitive men in particular, I would like to begin our conversation with a personal anecdote.

When I first met you at the HSP workshop in Stockholm in 2015, I remember going to the dining room of the hotel on the second day of the workshop to have breakfast. The dining room was packed, and it was incredibly loud and noisy, with lots of people talking and children running around. I remember feeling quickly stressed and overstimulated, and then I saw that you were having breakfast with your husband next to me. I remember thinking, "How does she manage it in here? I wonder whether she feels overstimulated, too." I don't know whether you remember this particular moment, but I wanted to ask whether you did actually feel overstimulated.

ELAINE ARON: I certainly remember lots of situations like that. And I remember that room. I think when you're with another person, it's a little bit like a buffer. You're focused on that person so you don't hear as much, especially if it's a familiar person. I don't think that's true when you're with a stranger, but if it is someone you're with a lot, then you have the sense that you've been here before. Familiarity is calming. That's part of what makes attachment so nice.

But one also has to take a lot of downtime around that sort of stimulation, like traveling and being in noisy places. I try to avoid those situations as much as possible. That situation in the dining room was not as unpleasant as some of them, but I remember on that day it was crazy. And, yes, in fact, one morning we went to a different dining room and hid there, but then there was a huge family and they were having a party there, so . . . [laughs]

TF: One just can't escape it. I think being easily overstimulated is often experienced as the biggest drawback when it comes to being a highly sensitive person. You mentioned that familiarity helps and trying to avoid overstimulating situations helps too, but apart from that, what else do you do in those situations? Have your personal strategies to deal with overstimulation changed over the years?

EA: Yes, I have observed that, as we get older, sensitive people get smarter about overstimulation. They avoid it more successfully. And I think that has been part of my strategy, to realize what it will be like when I get there and to avoid it as much as possible. I can't avoid the breakfast room in a hotel always. I mean, I could order in, but that comes with its own issues: the person coming in, tipping them. So planning ahead is the best strategy for me.

If you're stuck in an overstimulating situation, then figure this is how the universe is working today and just go for it. I do think that if you can relax around the overstimulation, it makes it less troublesome. I say people love the sound of the raindrops trickling, but if it's a faucet, people don't like it. They don't like hearing the neighbors through the wall doing the dishes, but when it's your partner doing the dishes, then it's a lovely sound. So it's also our interpretation of overstimulation that can add to our discomfort. Of course, I often think, "I hate this. I can't stand it in here anymore." And then it does really overwhelm me. But if I can relax around the overstimulation, it gets better. The saying "the ocean can't escape its waves" comes to mind.

TF: It sounds like you've developed a variety of strategies when it comes to dealing with overstimulation over the years. And if they all fail, we need to practice acceptance.

Let's focus on highly sensitive men. My impression is that men struggle a lot when it comes to accepting being highly sensitive, probably more than women do. Why do you think that is?

EA: I think for the most part it's cultural. Men in countries like India or Thailand, I've heard, have no problem with being sensitive. It is admired. It is often not an issue in Western cultures with men who grow up in artistic households, or where parents value the sensitivity in them as something desirable in a boy. That is rare, though, and often, to some extent, countercultural. But that's what we need: little subcultures that give sensitive men a sense of their particular worth to the world.

For the most part, though, each culture likes certain aspects of their children and doesn't like other aspects of their children. So if you want all your boys to grow up to be warriors, you like them to be little warriors from the beginning. If you like all the girls to be pretty little princesses, they will grow up as little princesses. You are in trouble if you were not born a warrior or a princess, but are, instead, say, a guy wants to be a musician or a girl wants to be a racehorse jockey. Some parents will try to make their little would-be jockeys as pretty as they can and will try to make those artistic boys as tough as they can.

TF: You just mentioned the particular role of highly sensitive men in society and what you say points to how important it is for them to know their worth, to hear from others that their sensitivity is not shameful, but appreciated and liked, and an important part of them. I think that is what often doesn't happen. Being sensitive is not seen as the "masculine ideal" in the Western world, so sensitive men can quickly feel that their sensitivity is not wanted or is disliked by others. I find your idea that sensitive men can also lead other men in certain areas of life because of their sensitivity, very interesting. So it sounds like you believe that strategizing, advising, and moving culture forward are the functions highly sensitive men might have in a given society.

EA: Yes. I think in the past, the lawyers, schoolteachers, doctors, ministers of court, artists, writers, scientists were mostly sensitive people because there were already so many jobs for the others. There was so much manual work to be done or shopkeeping, and a lot of people were happy to do it. But we're losing those jobs. The nonsensitive people have moved into law, medicine, teaching, etcetera, and they have taken them over. I think to their detriment, because they're becoming much more about making money, which I think sensitive people don't tend towards worrying so much about.

There are many exceptions, of course. I hate making generalizations, but sensitive people tend to see the bigger picture. They need to have meaningful work. They are less likely to put monetary gain at the top of their list of what's important for them. Of course, I'm uncomfortable making these kind of stereotypes. It's not a judgment, because we need money in the world, too. We need people to accumulate wealth, too, it seems. But it is trickier now for sensitive people to find meaningful work in their traditional fields when they do not feel empowered and appreciated for what they bring to law, to medicine, or to teaching. Or empowered to protect themselves from the inevitable overstimulation.

I remember a sensitive teacher I met who wanted to quit her job. "This is too much for me! I have to work 24–7 to do a good job." And I knew she was an excellent teacher. My own son had been in her class. So I said, "Do you think the kids would be better off if you do less or if you quit?" So she developed ways to make teaching less difficult for her. She was the envy of her colleagues because she always quit at four o'clock, she never took work home, and she had the kids grade their own papers. In other words, she found inventive ways of dealing with her sensitivity. Some people admired her; some people thought she was lazy. When she thought about it, she simply had to find a way to do her job as a sensitive person.

TF: We're now touching upon challenges highly sensitive people face in the work context; I know that there are whole books on this topic.[2]

When I spoke with highly sensitive men in preparation for this book, my impression was that finding one's niche or changing aspects of one's work so that it suits one's sensitive temperament is crucial. Of course, this is not always possible, but having worked on this with clients, it is often more possible than one might think. I've seen how much implementing little behavioral changes, like leaving on time or taking one's lunch break in a quiet setting, can make a huge difference. Only then can highly sensitive people thrive in their jobs and become able to use their sensitivity to the benefit of their job and themselves.

Of course, to implement change takes courage. When I spoke to highly sensitive men for this book, I was surprised to hear that most of them seemed to have found often very creative ways to change their job to suit their sensitivity. I almost expected this to be a bigger problem for them, but maybe this is where being a good strategist comes into play. However, what they did often perceive as problem-atic was that they felt a man is not allowed to be emotional. Whether that's at work or at home. And, of course, highly sensitive men are more emotional than other men.

This made me think about how radical it still seems for a man to be emotional or to show emotions openly to others, except anger, of course. No one is surprised by an angry man. He is easy to place; we're used to him. But a nervous, unsure, sad, fearful, or lonely man? A man who shows his feelings in front of others, speaks about them, or cries even? That seems to fit as badly as ever with the dominant image of what a man is meant to be.

What is your impression? Has it become easier for men to show emotions to others in the last ten or twenty years, or are we only say-ing it's easier for them, but actually, deep down inside we still reject the idea of an emotional man?

EA: My answer wouldn't be based on research; it would be based on observation. In the media, there seems to be a new enthusiasm for the "nerdy" guy. It seems like these guys are allowed to have more emotions.

At the same time, women are a little tired of men who show no emotions. You pick that up in the culture. Women always want everything: a tough guy who is deeply sensitive. They don't get both, so they may choose the very "manly" guy and then begin to realize, "I can't have any discussions with this guy that involve emotions. He just doesn't get it. He doesn't understand me or himself. I'm tired of having to teach him all the time." I think some people are picking up on it being an issue that men often have a hard time with emotions and that that is to the detriment of everyone around them.

Men who do show emotions are sometimes more valued because we do seem to be switching to a culture where close relationships often represent the meaning of life for many people. They don't know whether they have any religious beliefs anymore, but having a partner and children is the place in which you find the meaning of your life. Get ahead, yes, but once you got ahead, what do you have? It's like in movies about the guy who gets ahead, but then realizes it was all meaningless because he doesn't have any close relationships.

It seems like we're putting more value on close relationships, and there you need people who can get in touch with their feelings and show vulnerability in order to have closeness. So I think there is a shift in this direction.

TF: The idea that you need to be in touch with your own feelings and you need to show vulnerability to others in order to create real closeness or intimacy with—I think that is something that so many people struggle with.

If a highly sensitive man is brave enough to take risks or to make the first step, I think they are very good at forming close, intimate relationships with others. I get the sense it actually comes very easily to them, but they have to jump that first hurdle in order to do so. Some of the men I interviewed pointed out that they are very good at forming close relationships with men and women, but often feel that women put them in the "friend category" rather than in the "partner category."

What would you say to a woman who doesn't want to go for the sensitive guy because she thinks he is "too soft" or not exciting enough?

EA: Well, what I want to say is "You're a fool!" [laughs] Again, so many women talk about how they just can't have an intimate conversation with their husbands because they don't know how to do it. The problem is that, not all men, but many men have trouble identifying feelings, recognizing feelings, having empathy for others. It kind of makes sense, evolutionarily speaking, that if you have to kill another man, you don't want to be in touch with your feelings. If you're out there in the battlefield, fighting off the other guy, it's better not to feel a thing. But that's not the kind of person we need in the future. Clearly, in order to get along in a peaceful way, we need to have more empathy for each other. Not just be better at being cold-blooded, ruthless killers, which we have enough of as it is. I think empathy is a quality we want more of, and sensitive men have it.

TF: Let's stay with the topic of romantic relationships. Which skills, in your opinion, are important for highly sensitive men to have, apart from the ones we mentioned at the beginning of our conversation, to regulate their emotions or their level of overarousal in romantic relationships? I'm thinking here of how one deals with overstimulation, but also how we regulate our emotions in our relationship with our partner.

EA: I always divide it up into avoidance, endurance during overstimulation, and recovery afterwards. In a relationship, the challenge is always having the other person understand when you need downtime and to be alone, that it's not personal. It doesn't have anything to do with not liking them. You simply need time to yourself, some solitude, not talking, something like that. That's probably the main skill.

And saying no to some, not all, of the things that the other person might want to do that the sensitive man finds overstimulating—big parties, shopping malls, loud concerts, or sporting events. The only real problem with being highly sensitive is this overstimulation problem, and once you get that down and your partner understands that you are better company and more loving if you get some downtime, too, things are a lot easier.

What came to my mind before when we focused on the relationship between men and women is that a lot of it has to do with self-confidence. Because a lot of the men feel that there is something wrong with them if they are sensitive. As long as they're carrying this feeling of inferiority around with them, that's what women are likely to respond to. "I guess I have an inferior partner if even he thinks so." If a sensitive man feels like "I know what I'm doing here"—this kind of confidence, that they have better strategies, or that they can think things through, or know what they want and expect to get it or at least negotiate well—when you have that kind of confidence, I think that is very attractive.

Another issue that I keep running into with sensitive men is that they tend to be very cautious when it comes to making the first move. My husband—the social psychologist Art Aron—and I have done a lot of research on love and relationships. One of the things that we found early on was when people were asked what caused them to fall in love with the other person, it was when they found out the other person liked them. So sensitive men are cautious, which we all are, but especially sensitive people, we are cautious about doing something risky and may wait too long to act.

When we don't do something, that's a decision in itself. Like not having children. If you wait too long, you've made your decision by not deciding. You can wait too long with someone you're in love with, hoping that maybe you'll see a sign that they like you. Maybe you are worrying that they are not ready yet—they've been through a divorce, they're too young, etcetera—and then somebody else gets them while you're waiting for them to be ready. Again, a lot of that is a matter of confidence and being willing to take risks. It's important to realize that, if you fail, you do not need to feel completely devastated because you can feel positive about how you've tried, you acted. You've taken a risk; it didn't work out. Hey! Maybe it's the other person's problem. [laughs]

So I think confidence is the biggest problem for sensitive men and for the women who might be attracted to them. If the guy acts like he doesn't have confidence in himself, that's what's worrisome. I don't see any physical difference between sensitive and nonsensitive men. There may be small differences in how much muscle they have built

up because sensitive men may not be as interested in physical competition, but lots of them are hunks or into athletics or enjoy skiing
and hiking and all kinds of things, so it's not a question of appearance. If a woman wants a big muscular guy, she'll find a sensitive man
who is like that if that is what she wants. But those guys will also have
more confidence or self-confidence usually because they look less
sensitive to the rest of the world than they really are. Maybe most sensitive men should take up something physical that they can learn to
do well and makes them feel strong. I don't know. I had my sensitive
son learn judo. I did not know the term *sensitive*, but I recall the coach
saying to him when a smaller kid was holding him down, "Push him
off, just push him off." It was not in my son's nature. But he did have
more confidence around other boys because of a few tricks he learned
in judo. Never used them, but knew he had them. Maybe we should
have sport lessons just for sensitive boys.

This does mean that sensitive men have to work on confidence,
and that goes back to my first book: believing in their trait, knowing
it's *real* and knowing the good things about the trait. Not trying to
live like the other 80 percent, because if you're overaroused or overstimulated or exhausted, your mood won't be as good, your
confidence won't be as good.

Self-care is very important. It doesn't make you weak; it makes
you smart. Because your nervous system runs in a certain way, you
have to use that well. You can talk about the Porsche versus the
Chevrolet truck. You operate them differently. [laughs]

Being with other sensitive people is a big help, too. Knowing that
you belong to a group. It's just like coming out when you're gay. You
have to realize that there are other people like you that are strong
and proud and don't feel scared and weak. Then you have to heal
those old wounds, which we all carry to some degree, which affect
sensitive people more—that there's something wrong with us, which
is just not true. But we now know from differential susceptibility that
we can probably also heal better, benefitting from a good relationship. Healing doesn't mean it's gone, but it means we're smarter at

dealing with it. A sensitive person who lives "smart" is, I'm sure, attractive to other people.

TF: I think that is a very interesting point. The goal for a highly sensitive man should not be to become less sensitive or to live like a man who isn't highly sensitive. The goal has to be to become confidently sensitive. If you're able to develop a level of confidence about who you are as a highly sensitive man, if you manage to look after yourself, and if you're able to create a rich, deep, and meaningful life in which you flourish and have a good time, surely that is attractive to others, and in particular to potential romantic partners.

EA: Right. Exactly.

TF: Apart from what we just talked about, is there a key message you have for highly sensitive men who struggle with their confidence?

EA: Something that comes to mind is focusing on people who you know like you. There's got to be some people who like you because they think you're charming and wonderful and talented, interesting, or they just like you "for no reason"; you want to keep them in mind.

TF: So something that's both really practical, in that you can actually spend more time with these people, but also something that relates to how your see yourself. Like having an internalized support team that is cheering you on or speaks kindly to you in difficult moments.

EA: Yes. Nobody likes everybody; nobody is loved by everybody. Keep close to you the people with whom you feel love, and then carry them with you when you're out in the world where it doesn't seem like everybody loves you. Just remember them. I think it's important to keep love there, not just because it's nice to feel loved, but because it gives you confidence to know that, for some people at least, you're wonderful and charming and interesting. And for other people you will be, too. And the people that are not interested in you, well, it doesn't matter. They don't like Porsches; they like trucks. [laughs] Fine. Whatever you like. But there are people who really like you.

I love this little thing that I discovered when I was writing *The Undervalued Self* [2010]. I asked people to write a list of the people they feel good about being with and the people that make them uncomfortable. The people on the feel-good list they "linked" with—there was wanting to be around each other, wanting to know more about each other, wanting to help each other if you can. The people on the feel-bad list are those you rank yourself against. You're in comparison mode. Even when they think you're superior to them. You don't really like being with someone if they put you on a pedestal all the time. We have to compare and rank, but the less of it, the better.

TF: Yes, I think that is very important to remember. Not everybody has to like you. That's all right. But we can use the people who do know and like us as a source of comfort and support, as a shield when things become tricky.

When we talk about relationships, we must also think about non-romantic relationships, such as the relationships between fathers and their children. A topic that has come up in the research for this book is being a highly sensitive dad. Apart from finding ways to deal with overstimulation, what else do you think they need to consider in particular?

EA: Well, the thing with highly sensitive parents—and it applies to mothers and fathers alike—is that you're really, really good if you're not overstimulated. And if you're overstimulated, you're not very sensitive. You're miserable. So you've got to find a way to get enough help. But it can't just all fall on your partner. You've got to find ways to make it easier. It might be changing things at work so that you're not overtired at home. It may be hiring some help to run the house, if there isn't any. In other words, cutting down on the work, on the stimulation that goes with having children. You just have to do that. Because then you'll be more in tune than others with your child.

We did do a little survey of parents, mothers and fathers, though we didn't get as many fathers to respond as mothers. However, we did find that sensitive fathers, again like the mothers, found parenting harder and more stressful than other parents. But they were also more in tune with their children. Although the sample wasn't large enough to be completely reliable, we did find that sensitive fathers are probably particularly good when times get rough. Which they can in families.

TF: Why do you think highly sensitive fathers are particularly good in those situations?

EA: Well, let's say there is a death, or there isn't enough money. The sensitive fathers are more likely to be aware of how this is affecting the children. As opposed to the less sensitive father, who will go out and fight that problem. Get that job or do whatever is necessary. Like when you're hunting a mammoth and you can't think about the guy next to you falling or you can't be worried about whether your wife's delivery of the baby is going well because you've got to be focused on killing the mammoth. But if you're sensitive, you're going to have the bigger perspective, and you're going to take into account the fact that, not only do I have to get food on the table, but I also have to keep this from traumatizing my children.

So highly sensitive fathers are probably better at doing the emotional caregiving in the family, which we know now is the basis of so much. Whether the human race is a success or failure depends on how parents are responding to their children. It's not about survival anymore. It's much more about secure attachments. If the mother is constantly having to protect her children from the father's insensitivity, it just doesn't go well. Children need a lot of role modeling about how to be in the world, which is traditionally the role of the male. And if sensitivity, thoughtfulness, reflection, good strategizing, and all that are role modeled, then children go out in the world wiser and more successful.

If you think about the direction the world is going, if it's not going into free fall, it's going to be because of the traits that sensitive people have in abundance. Not that they are the only ones who think deeply or the only ones that have strong feelings, but those are the traits that are really going to matter in terms of the success of the planet. It's not the ability to kill mammoths, or to kill the enemy, or to do hard manual labor. It's subtlety.

TF: I think that's why the whole topic is so incredibly current. I can't help thinking that the characteristics and attributes that we associate with sensitive men, like compassion, the ability to find good strategies and solutions, are exactly what we need more of at the moment. An antidote to this destructive masculinity.

EA: Yes. And then the tricky thing is what can the sensitive men do for and about the less sensitive men? Not just never again getting bullied by those "mean boys." What can that kid, when he grows up, do to help the boys who are less sensitive, the men who are less sensitive? What strategies can a sensitive man develop? If you're dealing with kids that have not learned long division, you can't teach them algebra. So if you've got men who just don't think in certain ways, how do you get them to think a little bit more in that way without shaming them? Because if you shame them, they can turn around and shame you. Call you names, ridicule your way of living or being. So how do we work together?

I really think that sensitive peoples are really good at strategy, so it's kind of up to us to strategize. How to make changes in the other 80 percent without being self-righteous, which is almost impossible. And again, it's a question of superiority and inferiority. If we just could get away from it more!

TF: I wonder whether it comes back to the confidence issue we talked about earlier. If you're a highly sensitive man who feels confident, not in an arrogant way, but confident about his emotional needs, his worth and his boundaries, and you have friendships with men who aren't highly sensitive, you probably enable them to experience a significant amount of closeness and depth that they probably don't experience in their friendships with other non–highly sensitive people.

When a highly sensitive man is friends with a man who is less sensitive, then this less sensitive man is probably going to experience a significant amount of emotional openness, closeness, and depth that he probably isn't getting from his relationships with other men. And at the end of the day, this is something really special and valuable because deep down we're all searching for intimacy, a feeling of closeness and safety with other people, even if it can also trigger a sense of fear in us, and thus our defense mechanisms. But also, the highly sensitive man will experience a huge amount in this relationship that he, in turn, might not get from another highly sensitive man. In other words, I think this is also about recognizing and valuing what you as a sensitive man have to offer other people, precisely because of your high sensitivity.

EA: That's it. You got it! And it makes me think of the book *The Highly Sensitive Person in Love* and the interactions my husband and I had when I first wrote *The Highly Sensitive Person*. In the chapter on relationships, I wrote about how fortunate it can be for a highly sensitive person to be with a less sensitive partner because that person can do all the things that you can't. And then my husband read it and said, "You don't get it! You don't get how much I gain by being with you." So then we began to see the advantages and the disadvantages of these kinds of "mixed" relationships (and the odds are that about 50 percent of couples will be).

The first task really would be for the sensitive person to let the nonsensitive person see the advantages of being sensitive so that you do not feel one down. With my husband, I'm famous for picking the good hikes and the good restaurants because I remember details that he doesn't. He says, "Let's go back there." I say, "You don't remember that you hated the food there last time?" or "Remember they changed owners?" or "That's a great hike, but we don't want to go up there on a hot day." You get appreciated for that if you trust your own opinion. And you will after enough bad meals and hot hikes! [laughs]

But on the other hand, I can't make decisions, and he can make the decision. He can make a lot more arrangements and phone calls and do more administrative work than I can tolerate. The things that get overstimulating for me may be bothersome to him, but they don't get him down as quickly. The bottom line is: different, but just as good.

TF: Different, but just as good! I really like that. And I think that is something we can apply to all the friendships or relationships between highly sensitive people and those people who aren't highly sensitive.

EA: Tom, I think we're getting at something very neat here. You know the whole idea of a secure attachment style? The simple definition of a secure attachment style is that you generally like other people and you expect them to like you. Now, if you could go into the world as a sensitive person with the attitude, I generally like people who are not highly sensitive and they generally like me, how does that work? How do you get to that place? Well, through experiences in which you came to know that this really can work well. And then sort of spreading that into the world.

TF: Yes. I think that, as a highly sensitive man, developing this kind of attitude could change the way you feel in life and really open up new ways of behaving.

Elaine, is there anything else you would like to say about highly sensitive men before we end our conversation?

EA: Yes. Maybe something kind of personal. If I could have a second romantic partner, which I do not want, of course, because I have a wonderful husband, even if he is not highly sensitive, but if I could, it would be a highly sensitive man. I admire sensitive men—love them, I guess, as a group, those I have met—and want to cheer them on for what they can do for the world. We sensitive people are not superior, but we certainly are key members of the human team. Essential. Sensitive men especially.

TF: Thank you so much for this conversation!

Endnotes

Unless otherwise stated, all translations from German into English are the translator's own.

Epigraph: Jung, C. G. (2015). *Freud and Psychoanalysis*, (trans. Hull, R. F. C.). Vol. 4, London: Routledge, para. 398 and 399.

Introduction

1. Aron, E., and A. Aron. 1997. "Sensory Processing Sensitivity and Its Relation to Introversion and Emotionality." *Journal of Personality and Social Psychology* 73: 345–68.
2. Twenge, J. M., and W. K. Campbell. 2010. *The Narcissism Epidemic: Living in the Age of Entitlement.* New York: Atria Books.
3. Maaz, H.-J. 2014. *Die Narzisstische Gesellschaft—Ein Psychogramm.* Munich: dtv Verlagsgesellschaft.

Chapter 1: A Turning Point in Masculinity

1. Jardine, A. 2005. "Männer in der Krise: Jetzt reißt euch mal zusammen!" Brigitte, May 11. www.brigitte.de/liebe/beziehung/maenner-in-der-krise-537719/ (accessed April 24, 2017).
2. Raether, E., and T. Stelzer. 2014. "Das geschwächte Geschlecht." *Zeit Online*, January 2. www.zeit.de/2014/02/maenner-krise-maennerbewegung (accessed April 24, 2017).

3. Ehgoetz, S. [n.d.] "Wo ist das starke Geschlecht?" *Amica*. www.amica.de/ liebe-psychologie/psychotests/maennerkrise/maenner-krise-wo-ist-das-starke-geschlecht_aid_1919.html (accessed April 24, 2017).

4. Mieth, J. 2011. "Identitätssuche zwischen Super-Dad und eitlem Gockel." *Welt*, October 3. www.welt.de/lifestyle/article13639086/Identitaetssuche-zwischen-Super-Dad-und-eitlem-Gockel.html (accessed April 24, 2017).

5. *Psychologist* 27 (June 2014).

6. *BBC News*. 2013. "Diane Abbott to Warn of British 'Masculinity' Crisis." May 15. www.bbc.co.uk/news/uk-22530184 (accessed April 24 2017).

7. Marcotte, A. 2016. "Overcompensation Nation: It's Time to Admit That Toxic Masculinity Drives Gun Violence." *Salon*, June 3. www.salon.com/ 2016/06/13/overcompensation_nation_its_time_to_admit_that_toxic _masculinity_drives_gun_violence/ (accessed April 24, 2017).

8. Zimbardo, P., and N. D. Coulombe. 2015. Man Disconnected: How Technology Has Sabotaged What It Means to Be Male. London: Ryder.

9. Urwin, J. 2016. *Man Up—Surviving Modern Masculinity*. London: Icon Books.

10. Stokowski, M. 2016. "Es ist ein Junge." *Spiegel Online*, June 14, 2016. www.spiegel.de/kultur/gesellschaft/gewalt-der-taeter-ist-fast-immer -ein-mann-kolumne-a-1097493.html (accessed April 24, 2017).

11. Frosh, S., A. Phoenix, and R. Pattman. 2002. *Young Masculinities— Understanding Boys in Contemporary Society*. London: Palgrave Macmillan.

12. Thiele, A. 2002. "Gibt es eigentlich 'typisch männlich'? Rollenorientierung und männliche Hormone—Ergebnisse aus der psychologischen Männergesundheitsforschung." *Forschung Frankfurt* 1/2: 53–54.

13. Addis, M. E. 2008. "Gender and Depression in Men." *Clinical Psychology: Science and Practice* 15: 153–68.

14. Barker, Gary. 2018. "Why Do So Many Men Die by Suicide?" *Slate*, June 28. slate.com/human-interest/2018/06/are-we-socializing-men-to-die-by-suicide.html (accessed February 6, 2019).

15. National Institute on Drug Abuse. "Sex and Gender Differences in Drug Abuse." www.drugabuse.gov/publications/research-reports/substance-use-in-women/sex-gender-differences-in-substance-use (accessed February 6, 2019).

16. World Health Organization. 2000. "Fact Sheet No. 248, Women and Mental Health." www.who.int/mediacentre/factsheets/en (accessed April 24, 2017).

17. Mieth, Von Julian. 2011. "Identitätssuche zwischen Super-Dad und eitlem Gockel." Welt, October 3. www.welt.de/lifestyle/article13639086/

Identitaetssuche-zwischen-Super-Dad-und-eitlem-Gockel.html (accessed February 6, 2019).

18. 2018. "Undergraduate Retention and Graduation Rates." nces.ed.gov/programs/coe/pdf/coe_ctr.pdf (accessed February 6, 2019).

19. 2018. "Undergraduate Retention and Graduation Rates." nces.ed.gov/programs/coe/pdf/coe_ctr.pdf (accessed February 6, 2019).

20. Blue, L. 2008. "Why Do Women Live Longer Than Men?" *Time*, August 6, 2008. content.time.com/time/health/article/0,8599,1827162,00.html (accessed April 24, 2017).

21. Luy, M. 2011. "Ursachen der Geschlechterdifferenz in der Lebenser- wartung. Erkenntnisse aus der Klosterstudie." *Schweizerisches Medizin-Forum* 11, no. 35: 580–83.

22. Parker, Kim, and Gretchen Livingston. 2018. "7 Facts About American Dads." Pew Research Center, June 13. www.pewresearch.org/fact- tank/2018/06/13/fathers-day-facts/ (accessed February 6, 2019).

23. Addis, M. E., and J. R. Mahalik. 2003. "Men, Masculinity, and the Con- texts of Help Seeking." *American Psychologist* 58, no. 1: 5–14.

24. Good, G. E., T. S. Borst, and D. L. Wallace. 1994. "Masculinity Research: A Review and Critique." *Applied and Preventive Psychology* 3: 3–14.

25. Pleck, J. 1995. "The Gender Role Strain Paradigm: An Update." In R. Levant and W. Pollack, eds. *New Psychology of Men*. New York: Basic.

26. O'Neil, J. 2008. "Summarizing 25 Years of Research on Men's Gender Role Conflict Using the Gender Role Conflict Scale: New Research Par- adigms and Clinical Implications." *Counseling Psychologist* 38: 358–445.

27. Addis, M. E. 2008. "Gender and Depression in Men." *Clinical Psychology: Science and Practice* 15: 153–68.

28. O'Neil, J. 2008. Op. cit.

29. Haggett, A. 2015. *A History of Male Psychological Illness in Britain: 1945– 1980*. London: Palgrave Macmillan.

30. Micale, M. 2008. *Hysterical Men: The Hidden History of Male Nervous Ill- ness*. London: Harvard University Press.

31. Germer, C. 2009. *The Mindful Path to Self-Compassion: Freeing Yourself from Destructive Thoughts and Emotions*. New York: Guilford Press.

Chapter 2: Understanding High Sensitivity

1. Schneider, S. 2003. *Angststörungen bei Kindern und Jugendlichen: Grundla- gen und Behandlung*. Trossingen, Germany: Springer Verlag.

2. Oerter, R., and L. Montada, L., eds. 2008. *Entwicklungspsychologie*. Weinheim, Germany: Beltz.
3. Jung, C. G. 1976. *Psychological Types (The Collected Works of C. G. Jung, Vol. 6* [Bollingen Series XX]), Princeton, N.J.: Princeton University Press.
4. Eysenck, H. J., and S. B. G. Eysenck. 1968. *Manual for the Eysenck Personality Inventory*. San Diego, Calif.: Educational and Industrial Testing Service.
5. Schneider, S. 2003. *Angststörungen bei Kindern und Jugendlichen: Grundlagen und Behandlung*. Trossingen, Germany: Springer Verlag, 65.
6. Kristal, J. 2005. *The Temperament Perspective: Working With Children's Styles*. Baltimore, Md.: Brookes Publishing.
7. Lohaus, A., and M. Vierhaus. 2015. *Entwicklungspsychologie des Kindes- und Jugendalters für Bachelor*. Berlin: Springer Verlag.
8. Siegler, R., J. DeLoache, and N. Eisenberg. 2005. *Entwicklungspsychologie im Kindes- und Jugendalter*. Wiesbaden, Germany: Springer Spektrum.
9. Aron, E. N., A. Aron, and K. Davies. 2005. "Adult Shyness: The Interaction of Temperamental Sensitivity and an Adverse Childhood Environment." *Personality and Social Psychology Bulletin* 31: 181–97.
10. Stemmler, D., D. Hagemann, M. Amelang, and F. Spinath. 2016. *Differentielle Psychologie und Persönlichkeitsforschung*. Stuttgart, Germany: Kohlhammer Verlag.
11. Wolf, M., S. Van Doorn, and F. J. Weissing. 2008. "Evolutionary Emergence of Responsive and Unresponsive Personalities." *Proceedings of the National Academy of Sciences* 105, no. 41: 15, 825–30.
12. Pluess, M. 2015. "Individual Differences in Environmental Sensitivity." *Child Development Perspectives* 9: 1–6.
13. Belsky, J., M. J. Bakermans-Kranenburg, and M. H. van IJzendoorn. 2007. "For Better and for Worse. Differential Susceptibility to Environmental Influences." *Current Directions in Psychological Science* 16, no. 6: 300–304.
14. Belsky, J., and M. Pluess. 2009. "Beyond Diathesis Stress: Differential Susceptibility to Environmental Influences." *Psychological Bulletin* 135, no. 6: 885–908.
15. Ellis, B. J., and W. T. Boyce. 2008. "Biological Sensitivity to Context." *Current Directions in Psychological Science* 17, no. 3: 183–87.
16. Glomp, I. 2011. "Glücksfall Problemkind." *Bild der Wissenschaft*, 84–86. www.wissenschaft.de/gesellschaft-psychologie/gluecksfall-problemkind (accessed February 6, 2019).
17. Jagiellowicz, J., X. Xu, A. Aron, E. Aron, G. Cao, T. Feng, and X. Weng. 2010. "The Trait of Sensory Processing Sensitivity and Neural Re-

sponses to Changes in Visual Scenes." *Social Cognitive and Affective Neuroscience* 6: 38–47.

18. Pluess, M. and I. Boniwell. 2015. "Sensory-Processing Sensitivity Predicts Treatment Response to a School-Based Depression Prevention Program: Evidence of Vantage Sensitivity." *Personality and Individual Differences* 82: 40–45.

19. Bianca P. B. Acevedo, E. Aron, A. Aron, M. Sangster, N. Collins, and L. Brown. 2014. "The Highly Sensitive Brain: An fMRI Study of Sensory Processing Sensitivity and Response to Others' Emotions." *Brain and Behavior* 4: 580–94.

20. Lionnetti, F., A. Aron, E. N. Aron, G. L. Burns, J. Jagiellowicz, and M. Pluess. 2018. "Dandelions, Tulips and Orchids: Evidence for the Existence of Low-Sensitive, Medium-Sensitive, and High-Sensitive Individuals." *Translational Psychiatry* 8, no. 1: 24.

21. Aron, E. 2010. *Psychotherapy and the Highly Sensitive Person.* New York: Routledge.

22. Ibid.

23. Zuckerman, M. 1988. "Behavior and Biology: Research on Sensation Seeking and Reactions to the Media." In L. Donohew, H. E. Sypher, and E. T. Higgins, eds. *Communication, Social Cognition and Affect.* Hillsdale, N.J.: Lawrence Erlbaum.

24. Zuckerman, M. "The Genetic Basis of Risk-Seeking." 2012. bigthink.com. www.youtube.com/watch?v=oWk3lSIXmPE (accessed June 6, 2017).

25. Aron, E. 2010. *Psychotherapy and the Highly Sensitive Person.* New York: Routledge.

26. Aron, E. 2001. *The Highly Sensitive Person in Love: Understanding and Managing Relationships When the World Overwhelms You.* New York: Harmony.

27. Pluess, M. 2017. "Vantage Sensitivity: Environmental Sensitivity to Positive Experiences as a Function of Genetic Differences." *Journal of Personality* 85, no. 1: 38–50.

Chapter 3: Identifying High Sensitivity

1. Aron, E. 2010. *Psychotherapy and the Highly Sensitive Person.* New York: Routledge.

2. Yerkes, R. M., and J. D. Dodson. 1908. "The Relation of Strength of Stimulus to Rapidity of Habit-Formation." *Journal of Comparative Neurology and Psychology* 18: 459–82.

3. Melamed, S., U. Ugarten, A. Shirom, L. Kahana, Y. Lerman, and P. Froom. 1999. "Chronic Burnout, Somatic Arousal and Elevated Salivary Cortisol Levels." *Journal of Psychosomatic Research* 46, no. 6: 591–98.

4. Lammers, C.-H. 2015. *Emotionsfokussierte Methoden: Techniken der Verhaltenstherapie.* Weinheim, Germany: Beltz.

5. Aron, E. 2010. Op. cit.

Chapter 4: Everyday Effects of High Sensitivity and How It Differs from Psychological Disorders

1. Beisser, A. R. 1997. Die paradoxe Theorie der Veränderung. In A. R. Beisser, *Wozu brauche ich Flügel?—Ein Gestalttherapeut betrachtet sein Leben als Gelähmter.* Wuppertal, Germany: Hammer, 144–48.

2. *Internationale Klassifikation psychischer Störungen: ICD-10.* Kapitel V (F). Klinisch-diagnostische Leitlinien. Bern, Switzerland: Verlag Hans Huber.

3. Aron, E., A. Aron, and K. M. Davies. 2005. "Adult Shyness: The Interaction of Temperamental Sensitivity and an Adverse Childhood Environment." *Personality and Social Psychology Bulletin* 31: 181–97.

4. Hofmann, S., and S. Bitran. 2007. "Sensory-Processing Sensitivity in Social Anxiety Disorder: Relationship to Harm Avoidance and Diagnostic Subtypes." *Journal of Anxiety Disorders* 21, no. 7: 944–54.

5. *Internationale Klassifikation psychischer Störungen: ICD-10.* Kapitel V (F). Klinisch-diagnostische Leitlinien. Bern, Switzerland: Verlag Hans Huber.

6. Ibid.

Chapter 5: Strategies to Deal With Overstimulation and Intense Emotions—What Emotional Regulation Is

1. Lammers, C.-H. 2015. *Emotionsfokussierte Methoden: Techniken der Verhaltenstherapie.* Weinheim, Germany: Beltz.

2. Brindle, K., R. Moulding, K. Bakker, and M. Nedeljkovic. 2015. "Is the Relationship Between Sensory-Processing Sensitivity and Negative Affect Mediated by Emotional Regulation?" *Australian Journal of Psychology* 67: 214–21.

3. Ekman, P. 2007. *Emotions Revealed, Second Edition: Recognizing Faces and Feelings to Improve Communication and Emotional Life*. New York: Henry Holt. Ekman later added four further emotions to this original list of seven.

4. Lammers, C.-H. 2015. *Emotionsfokussierte Methoden: Techniken der Verhaltenstherapie*. Weinheim, Germany: Beltz.

5. Grawe, K. 2000. *Psychologische Therapie*. Göttingen, Germany: Hogrefe.

6. Lammers, C.-H. 2011. *Emotionsbezogene Psychotherapie—Grundlagen, Strategien und Techniken*. Stuttgart, Germany: Schattauer.

Chapter 6: Strategies to Deal With Overstimulation and Intense Emotions—Mindfulness and Acceptance

1. Lammers, C.-H. 2011. *Emotionsbezogene Psychotherapie—Grundlagen, Strategien und Techniken*. Stuttgart, Germany: Schattauer.

2. Ibid.

3. Brown, K. W., and R. M. Ryan. 2003. "The Benefits of Being Present: Mindfulness and Its Role in Psychological Well-Being." *Journal of Personality and Social Psychology* 84, no. 4: 822–48.

4. Michalak, J., T. Heidenreich, and J. M. G. Williams. 2012. *Achtsamkeit*. Göttingen, Germany: Hogrefe.

5. Chozen Bays, J. 2011. *How to Train a Wild Elephant: And Other Adventures in Mindfulness*. Boulder, Colo.: Shambhala Publications.

6. Hayes, S. C. 2005. *Get Out of Your Mind and Into Your Life: The New Acceptance and Commitment Therapy*. Oakland, Calif.: New Harbinger Publications.

Chapter 7: Strategies to Deal With Overstimulation and Intense Emotions—Relaxation and Imagery Exercises

1. Reddemann, L. 2005. *Imagination als heilsame Kraft*. Stuttgart, Germany: Klett-Cotta.

Chapter 8: Your Relationship with Yourself

1. Lockard, A. J., J. A. Hayes, K. Neff, and B. D. Locke. 2014. "Self-Compassion Among College Counseling Center Clients: An Examination

of Clinical Norms and Group Differences." *Journal of College Counseling* 17: 249–59.

2. Gilbert, P. 2009. "Introducing Compassion-Focused Therapy." *Advances in Psychiatric Treatment* 15, no. 3: 199–208.

3. Breines, J. G., and S. Chen. 2012. "Self-Compassion Increases Self-Improvement Motivation." *Personality and Social Psychology Bulletin* 38, no. 9: 133–43.

4. Brähler, C. 2016. *Selbstmitgefühl entwickeln—liebevoller werden mit sich selbst.* Munich: Scorpio Verlag.

5. Gilbert, P. 2013. *Compassion Focused Therapy.* Paderborn, Germany: Junfermann Verlag.

6. Ibid.

7. Ibid.

8. Peichl, J. 2011. *Jedes Ich ist viele Teile—Die inneren Selbst-Anteile als Ressource nutzen.* Munich: Kösel.

Chapter 9: Self-Worth and Self-Care for Highly Sensitive Men

1. Baumeister, R. F., L. Smart, and J. M. Boden. 1996. "Relation of Threatened Egotism to Violence and Aggression: The Dark Side of High Self-Esteem." *Psychological Review* 103, no. 1: 5–33.

2. Stucke, T. S., and S. L. Sporer. 2002. "When a Grandiose Self-Image Is Threatened: Narcissism and Self-Concept Clarity as Predictors for Negative Emotions and Aggression Following Ego Threat." *Journal of Personality* 70: 509–32.

3. Crocker, J., and L. E. Park. 2004. "The Costly Pursuit of Self-Esteem." *Psychological Bulletin* 130, no. 3: 392–414.

4. Orth, U., J. Maes, and M. Schmitt. 2015. "Self-Esteem Development Across the Life Span: A Longitudinal Study With a Large Sample From Germany." *Developmental Psychology* 51: 248–59.

5. Potreck-Rose, F., and G. Jacob. 2008. *Selbstzuwendung, Selbstakzeptanz, Selbstvertrauen—Psychotherapeutische Interventionen zum Aufbau von Selbstwertgefühl.* Stuttgart, Germany: Klett-Cotta.

Appendix: A Conversation with Elaine Aron About Highly Sensitive Men

1. Strohmaier, B. 2015. "Hochsensibilität ist keine Krankheit," *Welt*, March 1, 2015. www.welt.de/icon/article137874821/Hochsensibilitaet -ist-keine-Krankheit.html (accessed February 4, 2019).
2. Cooper, T. M. 2015. *Thrive! The Highly Sensitive Person and Career*. Ozark, Mo.: Invictus.

Acknowledgments

I WOULD LIKE TO THANK a number of important people who have accompanied me on this long journey and thus had a huge influence on this book. First and foremost, I want to thank Junfermann Verlag in Germany for their support and input, especially my German editor, Katharina Arnold. I couldn't have wished for a better editor! I would also like to extend my heartfelt thanks to my American editor, Denise Silvestro at Kensington, for her enthusiasm and hard work in putting together the English edition of this book. Thanks also to Ingrid Parlow in Vienna for her instant passion for this project when it was still just a sketch.

I would like to thank the following people who played an invaluable role in my research and in the journey of this book: Jamie Joseph, Linda Morison, Martin Seager, Mikael Gustafsson, Alison Haggett, Andrew Smiler, Tim Lomas, Christopher Germer, Ted Zeff, Georg Wißmann, Michael Ammann, Tara Cutland Green, and Brigitte Küster. Thanks are also due to translators Ben Fergusson (German to English) and Christa Broermann (English to German) for their excellent translations.

I owe special thanks to Michael Pluess for his friendly openness and all the time he's given me. And, of course, I would like to thank Elaine Aron from the bottom of my heart—for her research, for her generosity and warm support, and for her unique perspective on what it means to be a human being. All of these things have had a huge influence on both my life and my work as a psychotherapist over the past few years.

I would also like to thank my family and my friends: a particular thank you to Judith Hübner, Sara Zeugmann, and Valeska Falkenstein, who proofread early versions of this book and shared their invaluable feedback with me.

And, finally, I would like to thank all of the highly sensitive men who trusted me with their life stories, opening themselves up and showing me their humanity. They are all examples of a masculinity that combines strength, emotion, *and* sensitivity. Their strength and their belief in this book were the driving forces behind my writing and were genuinely indispensable.

Index

Mood swings, 81, 82
Mortality rates and gender, 14–15
Multitasking, 50, 54, 71, 164–65, 210
Music
    Darryl, 42–46
    high sensitivity to, 63, 64
    Sebastian, 214–18
    self-care strategies, 207

Narcissism, 5, 193
Narcissistic personality disorder,
    86–87
Natural selection, 37–38
Nature connectedness, 64, 206, 218
Neff, Kristin, 171–72, 173–74
Negative emotions, 59, 95, 97, 133,
    192
Neuroticism compared with high
    sensitivity, 40–41
"New man," 16

Oliver, 48–51, 52–53, 57–58, 60–61,
    210–11
O'Neil, Jim, 17–18
Orchid children, 37, 39, 97
Orientation and control, need for,
    102
Overstimulation, 50, 54–58, 76–77,
    93–94
    Aron on, 222–23
    arousal level and, 54–55, 57
    characteristics and behaviors,
        58
    cortisol levels and, 55–56
    of Darryl, 43
    DOES indicators, 50, 64, 65
    of Henry, 113
    of John, 25
    of Oliver, 57–58, 65
    of Peter, 69, 70

questions about typical prob-
    lem areas, 79–80
recognizing signs of, 99–101
strategies for dealing with. *See*
    Acceptance of feelings;
    Imagery exercises;
    Mindfulness; Physical
    relaxation
Overtime, 209

Pain threshold, 34
Parent-child bond, 30
Paternity leave, 16
Perfectionism, 43, 45–46, 53–54,
    123, 146
Perfume sensitivity, 49
Perls, Thomas, 15
Personality, 30–31
Personality disorders, 85–87
Physical relaxation, 96, 143–56
    body scan, 145–49
    in everyday life, 204–5, 207
    in everyday life, questionnaire,
        154–56
    progressive muscle relaxation,
        149–53
    at work, 211
Pleasure, 102, 113, 208
Pluess, Michael, 35–36, 39
Positive experiences and stimuli,
    208
Post-traumatic stress disorder
    (PTSD), 84–85
Potreck-Rose, Friederike, 195–96
Prefrontal cortex, 116–18
Present in the moment, 128–30
Progressive muscle relaxation
    (PMR), 149–53
Promiscuity, 25–26, 109, 111,
    112–13

About the Author

TOM FALKENSTEIN is a cognitive behavioral psychotherapist. After leaving school, he completed his German civilian service in Israel, and since 1999, he has worked in a variety of roles with people with psychological issues. After completing his degree in psychology in the United Kingdom, he completed his therapeutic training at the German Society for Behavioral Therapy in 2011. He then worked for a number of years as a psychotherapist in a general psychiatric clinic in London. It was during this time that he developed a particular interest in high sensitivity and therapeutic work with highly sensitive people and began to undertake training and supervision with Elaine Aron, Ph.D., author of *The Highly Sensitive Person*. He currently runs his own psychotherapeutic practice in Germany, and in 2015, he founded the European Centre for High Sensitivity (www.hsp-eu.com). The center is based in Berlin and offers consultations in both German and English for highly sensitive people.